ROJECT MANAGEMENT
OR THE ADVANCED
RACTICE NURSE

AROLYN SIPES

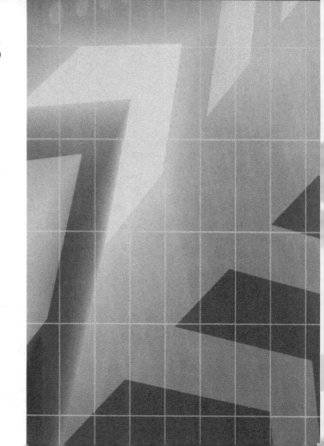

RINGER PUBLISHING COMPANY

Project Management for the
Advanced Practice Nurse

Carolyn Sipes, PhD, RN-BC, CNS, APN, PMP, is an associate professor at Chamberlain College of Nursing, and the subject matter expert (SME) for MSN Nursing Informatics Specialty Track. Dr. Sipes has more than 30 years' experience in management, as a director and in other nurse executive leadership positions, while also teaching part time. At the executive level, she worked as a consultant for implementations of electronic medical records (EMRs) at companies such as IBM, where she was involved in work on the iSOFT pilot project in England with the National Health System (NHS). It was here she achieved her project management professional (PMP) certification through the Project Management Institute (PMI). She also is board certified by the American Nurses Credentialing Center in Nursing Informatics (RN-BC) and holds a PhD, as well as clinical nurse specialist (CNS) and advanced practice nursing (APN) licenses. She also holds eight Epic certifications for clinical EHR implementations.

Dr. Sipes has worked as a senior/principal consultant on 23 EMR implementations over 12 years for such companies as HealthLink, Healthcare Informatics Associates, Inc. (HIA), Cleveland Clinic Abu Dhabi, to name a few. Dr. Sipes is the president, CEO, and founder of the Center for EHR Program Management, LLC, a consulting company for the implementations of EHRs.

Dr. Sipes started her nursing career as a BSN, working in neurology/neurosurgery, then completed her MSN and CNS while working in home care in Chicago, then as a pediatric AIDS CNS and as a NIH study coordinator for pediatric AIDS. She received an NIH fellowship to complete her doctoral studies in HIV/AIDS at Rush University, Chicago. During this time she also worked as a director of outcomes research and designed the Medical Outcomes System Assessment tool (MOS) used to evaluate physical functional assessments for subacute care organizations. Her dissertation on male caregivers who provided care for their partners with HIV/AIDS has been published and updated numerous times. During this time she also served as the vice president of an HIV/AIDs clinic in Chicago. After completing her doctorate, she worked as a research scientist for a major pharmaceutical company where she designed the Tolerability of Medication Assessment tool (TOMA). The research conducted using this tool was presented at the World AIDS Conference in Barcelona, Spain.

Dr. Sipes began designing and teaching informatics courses while consulting as a full-time senior project manager/director. These experiences led her to teaching informatics full time at the master's and doctoral levels. She has also published and presented, nationally and internationally, more than 19 nursing informatics and project management topics including webinars for the American Association of Colleges of Nursing, over the past 3 years.

Project Management for the Advanced Practice Nurse

Carolyn Sipes, PhD, RN-BC, CNS, APN, PMP

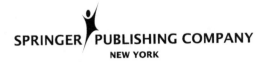

SPRINGER PUBLISHING COMPANY
NEW YORK

Springer Publishing Company, LLC
11 West 42nd Street
New York, NY 10036
www.springerpub.com

Acquisitions Editor: Joseph Morita
Composition: MPS Ltd, India

ISBN: 978-0-8261-2817-1
e-book ISBN: 978-0-8261-2818-8

15 16 17 18 / 5 4 3 2 1

The author and the publisher of this Work have made every effort to use sources believed to be reliable to provide information that is accurate and compatible with the standards generally accepted at the time of publication. Because medical science is continually advancing, our knowledge base continues to expand. Therefore, as new information becomes available, changes in procedures become necessary. We recommend that the reader always consult current research and specific institutional policies before performing any clinical procedure. The author and publisher shall not be liable for any special, consequential, or exemplary damages resulting, in whole or in part, from the readers' use of, or reliance on, the information contained in this book. The publisher has no responsibility for the persistence or accuracy of URLs for external or third-party Internet websites referred to in this publication and does not guarantee that any content on such websites is, or will remain, accurate or appropriate.

Library of Congress Cataloging-in-Publication Data
Sipes, Carolyn, author.
  Project management for the advanced practice nurse / Carolyn Sipes.
    p. ; cm.
  Includes bibliographical references and index.
  ISBN 978-0-8261-2817-1—ISBN 978-0-8261-2818-8 (e-book)
  I. Title.
  [DNLM: 1. Advanced Practice Nursing—organization & administration.
  2. Planning Techniques.   3. Program Development. WY 128]
  RT41
  610.73—dc23   2015016250

Printed in the United States of America by McNaughton & Gunn.

Contents

Section III: Application of Project Management Concepts and Tools

Foreword

Project management is an important skill in both career and life, yet little has been written to provide nurses and other health care professionals acting in leadership and advanced practice roles with the tools needed to ensure success in this area. The lack of literature and texts serves neither educators nor health care professionals well and has forced them to draw from other disciplines—until now, with the culmination of this book.

In part, the lack of project management literature may be attributed to its fairly recent definition as well as confusion over its defining characteristics and how those characteristics distinguish it from other aspects of management. According to the Project Management Institute (PMI), project management is "the application of knowledge, skills, tools, and techniques to project activities to meet the project requirements" (2008, p. 6). Project management consists of five phases—initiation, planning, implementing/executing, controlling, and closing. Projects differ from other activities because of their temporary nature and intent to create a unique product or service.

PMI also sought to establish project management as a profession, although it is not necessary to formally assume that role to benefit and apply associated knowledge and skills, as will be demonstrated through the many examples provided in this book. It is my contention that project management skills will play a key role in the collaborative transformation of the health care delivery system through the efforts of engaged health care professionals, payors, and consumers via a multitude of projects over time. *The Future of Nursing* report (Institute of Medicine [IOM], 2010) specifically calls for nurses to play a pivotal role in transformation. One tool to achieve transformation is information technology. The implementation of any information technology in a given health care organization exemplifies a project. Nursing informatics as a specialty delineates project management as key to its work. The American Nurses Credentialing Center (2013) test content outline for the informatics nursing credentialing examination includes content on all facets of project management. As a long-time nurse educator and co-author of *Handbook of Informatics for Nurses and Health Care Professionals,* I recognize the importance of project management to successful outcomes and particularly to the integration of information systems and technology.

This book offers guidance and insights and ties the skills of a seasoned project manager, advanced practice nurse, and nurse educator together to take the reader through all phases of the project management process from start to finish through tools integrated throughout the text.

Toni Hebda, PhD, RN-BC, MSIS, CNE
Professor, MSN Program
Chamberlain College of Nursing

REFERENCES

American Nurses Credentialing Center. (Last Update: 8/26/2013). Test Content Outline. Retrieved from http://www.nursecredentialing.org/Informatics-TCO2014 p. 4 of 5

Institute of Medicine (IOM). (2010). *The Future of Nursing: Leading Change, Advancing Health.* Washington, DC: The National Academies Press. Retrieved from http://books.nap.edu

Project Management Institute, Inc. (2008). *A guide to the project management body of knowledge (PMBOK Guide)* (4th ed.), p. 6. Newtown Square, PA: Project Management Institute, Inc.

Preface

The concept of this book grew from teaching nursing informatics and working as a consultant and project manager (PM) implementing electronic medical records. This author frequently noticed the lack of project management skills in nurses and other health care professionals; skills these professionals were expected to have and use. Nurses are greatly skilled at managing patient care and outcomes—processes that are similar to those used in project management—but they have failed to connect the dots, fearing they do not have the skills even when they are employing the organizational frameworks also used in project management. This book attempts to aid health care professionals in understanding and implementing project management. It outlines the phases of project management and offers tools that help one apply these skills.

This book is organized into three sections, following the convention of project management standards originally developed in the 1950s by engineers. Although based on proven concepts, this book is focused on defining those concepts in a way that nonproject managers, such as advanced practice nurses (APNs), doctors of nursing practice (DNPs), and other clinicians, can better comprehend so as to be able to apply definitions and processes used in the business operations side of a health care organization. Many tools used in management are included in each chapter. The first section is the introduction; APN role descriptions. The next section consists of the five basic concepts of project management, including the basics of monitoring timelines, a project's design and planning steps, implementation of the project plan, the monitoring and control phase, and the steps to take when closing a project. The final section provides exemplars of how current APNs and DNPs might use and apply project management skills using the various chapter toolkits as they implement a project at work or prepare a practicum assignment for graduation.

To be more specific, the following chapters provide many details outlining the expectations, tools, and deliverables needed for each of the steps of the project management process. For example, Chapter 1 includes the key concepts and definitions of the key skill areas an APN as PM should know. Constraints are defined, as are project steps. Chapter 2 lists some of the common roles an APN might assume and includes sample job descriptions for which project management skills are required. The design steps are found in Chapter 3, including descriptions of what to do first, such as gap and workflow analysis, team and system selection, work breakdown structure, creating a responsibility matrix, understanding team behaviors, and developing a project charter and scope, as well as other necessary management documents and tools. Chapter 4 includes the steps to take when developing a project plan, network diagram, risk management plan, communication plan, change management plan, kick-off meeting, and launching the project. Chapter 5 explains supervision and implementation, which comprise the longest phase in a project and include processes for implementing the plans developed in the previous steps. Status reports and tracking tools become a critical component of implementation, as do other elements of quality control such as testing and go-live processes. Chapter 6 describes the monitoring and control steps and defines the processes and tools needed to track the implementation, performance assessment, and dashboard reports, while controlling budgets and resources. Chapter 7 outlines the concluding and closing steps of the project management process and explains how to do the verification audit using the audit tool, how to conduct a lessons-learned assessment that verifies all processes are complete, how to arrange for postimplementation assessment and follow-up, and, finally, formal sign off by all steering committees, sponsors, stakeholders, and leadership. The final section includes exemplars of how and where the APN, DNP, chief nurse informatics officer (CNIO), clinical nurse specialist (CNS), nurse practitioner (NP), and others might apply concepts of project management to their everyday practice.

Carolyn Sipes

Acknowledgments

I am deeply grateful for the love, patience, continued encouragement, and support of my husband, Jim, and my family: Chris, Doug, and Susan, their husbands and wives, Jill and Rick, as well as toddler Josh.

I am also extremely grateful for the ongoing support and continued encouragement of peer faculty at Chamberlain College of Nursing: director of the MSN program, Dr. Kathleen Hunter, and professors Dr. Dee McGonigle and Dr. Toni Hebda. I could never have completed this project without their continued support.

Share

Project Management for the Advanced Practice Nu

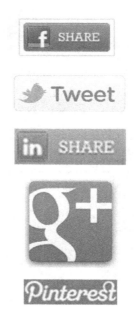

Introduction and Roles of the Advanced Practice Nurse

Basic Project Management for Advanced Practice Nurses and Health Care Professionals

LEARNING OBJECTIVES

Upon completion of this chapter, the reader will be able to:

1. Discuss three driving forces that develop project management skills
2. Discuss the history of project management
3. Discuss why project management is needed
4. List three principles of project management
5. List two tasks that program management addresses
6. Identify the constraints of project management outline

OUTLINE

- Key Terms
- Introduction
- Examples of APN Projects/Roles
- The Nursing Process and Project Management
- Definition of a Project
- What Is Project Management?
- Project Management Processes
- Principles of Project Management
- Project Management: Why Do We Need It?

KEY TERMS

American Association of Colleges of Nursing (AACN)

American Nurses Association (ANA)

Advanced practice nurse (APN)

Certified nurse-midwife (CNM)

Certified nursing specialist (CNS)

Certified registered nurse anesthetist (CRNA)

Chief nursing officer (CNO)

Doctor of nursing practice (DNP)

Electronic health record (EHR)

Informatics nurse specialist (INS)

Nurse administrator (NA)

Nurse informaticist (NI)

Nurse practitioner (NP)

Project manager (PM)

INTRODUCTION

Amy has been working on the medical floor of St. Joe's Hospital for 5 years and is in the master's of science in nursing (MSN) program at the local university where she has completed her core courses and is now taking the final management courses. The chief nursing officer (CNO) has learned of Amy's career goals and wants Amy to be considered for promotion to nurse manager of the medical department. The CNO reminds Amy that in addition to completing the management courses, she will also have to choose and develop a practicum project before she graduates. The prospect of the project makes Amy very nervous; she indicates that she does not know how to do a project and has never done one.

The CNO encourages Amy and reminds her how she helped organize her sister's wedding last summer; how she helped to set a date, plan who would be there, select the invitations, arrange for the church, and all of the other details that go into planning a wedding. The CNO says that her practicum will be a project with similar tasks, such as designing what she will do based on a health issue she would like to resolve. After this, Amy will then plan the necessary steps to complete the project, including setting end dates for completion, then after she has planned her project, will need to implement it step by step and finally assess her results and determine what will need to be fixed or changed.

The CNO assures Amy that completing the practicum is also a bit like the nursing process in that many of the five steps are the same for both processes—some of the terminology is different but the point is the same and follows the steps in the nursing process. She also reminds Amy that her project has a starting point and an end point, that it will be short term, unlike some of the endeavors the hospital has proposed that take years to complete. The CNO further assures Amy that she will be her mentor and that she has developed and implemented many projects in the past as part of her CNO training and current role responsibility. She will help Amy learn project management skills.

So, let us start with some of the basics Amy will need to learn. However, before we get into the basics of project management, it is important to first understand how the project management process will affect advanced practice nurses (APNs), such as Amy, and other health care professionals, such as the CNO. Chapters 1 and 2 define some of the key roles one assumes as project manager (PM) or when using some of the project management skills in practice. The concepts are based on proven project management standards and terminology developed over decades of practice. This chapter is focused on defining concepts in a way that non-project managers, such as APNs and other health care clinicians, will better understand in order to apply definitions and processes used in the business operations of a health care organization.

APNs will employ principles of project management for which they are uniquely suited, especially because they are particularly well suited for information technology (IT) implementations, as they essentially follow the nursing process of assessment, diagnosis, planning, implementation, and evaluation (American Nurses Association [ANA], 2008, 2010). In that sense, the APN can be viewed as the "manager" of patient care, applying similar processes to determine and achieve a specific outcome.

Chapter 1 is organized to define similarities between the nursing process and project management. Basic project management definitions, processes, concepts, and plans will be developed starting in Section II. Remember that project management is similar to the nursing process, as a project will be designed, planned, applied, carried out while being supervised, regulated, or controlled, and then finally, ended or concluded. Chapter 2 includes the different PM roles that might be assumed and applied by APNs.

Section II includes each of the five steps of project management, defined with a list of the activities that occur in that phase. It also includes examples of the tools that are used in each step as well as a description of the content that is used with the documents.

Section III contains Chapter 8, which provides case studies and exemplars that suggest how the APN, doctor of nursing practice (DNP), and other health care professionals will use different concepts of project management in different projects they might direct or when organizing a project they might need to develop for their doctorate of nursing practice. Different examples of project management are included for the role of APN as an administrator, certified nursing specialist (CNS), nurse practitioner (NP), chief nurse informatics officer (CNIO), or other levels of management in an organization.

EXAMPLES OF APN PROJECTS/ROLES

According to a report by the American Association of Colleges of Nursing (AACN), an APN can assume many different roles, including working as

- **Nurse practitioners (NP)** who deliver frontline primary and acute care in community clinics, schools, hospitals, and other settings, and perform such services as diagnosing and treating common acute illnesses and injuries, providing immunizations, conducting physical exams, and managing high blood pressure, diabetes, and other chronic problems.
- **Certified nurse-midwives (CNM)** who provide prenatal and gynecological care to normal healthy women; deliver babies in hospitals, private homes, and birthing centers; and continue with follow-up postpartum care.
- **Clinical nurse specialists (CNS)** who provide care in a range of specialty areas, such as cardiac, oncology, neonatal, pediatric, and obstetric/gynecologic nursing.
- **Certified registered nurse anesthetists (CRNA)** who administer more than 65% of all anesthetics given to patients each year and are the sole providers of anesthesia in approximately one third of U.S. hospitals (American Association of Colleges of Nursing [AACN], 2014).

These roles are ones that most frequently come to mind when considering an APN, but there are many others, and roles continue to be revised, updated, and expanded. Potential projects an APN might assume—that would require one to understand and use various project management skills—are included in the following sections.

Typically, an APN would use these skills to complete a graduate practicum that would need to be designed, planned, and implemented before graduation. Project management skills are discussed later and correlate to the nursing process. Examples of some of the projects an APN might consider would be:

- Evaluating a learning management system that has been implemented
- Assessing gaps in patients' needs and developing recommendations for practice
- Assessing the quality of how a particular process or program is functioning
- Mentoring other graduate students' development and recommending strategies for implementation of processes and programs to meet identified needs
- Designing qualitative tools to collect data
- Developing evidence-based practice guidelines for certain programs, such as wound management
- Developing and conducting a needs assessment for a population of patients
- Designing and implementing protocols for a hospital-wide program to address the identification, prevention, and treatment of skin tears

Examples of APN roles are listed in Table 1.1. This is a partial list and will change as APN roles are expanded and updated.

Table 1.1
Examples of Advanced Practice Nurse Roles

Nurse administrator (NA)
Nurse practitioner (NP)
Clinical nurse specialist (CNS)
Certified registered nurse anesthetist (CRNA)
Certified nurse-midwife (CNM)
Nurse informatist
Informatics nurse specialist (INS)
Doctor of nursing practice (DNP)
Director of advanced practice nursing

From Sipes (2014).

In addition to the examples listed in Table 1.1, DNPs maintain clinical practice, conduct program evaluations, implement practice changes and improvements, manage quality improvement, and translate evidence into practice. The difference between a PhD and DNP is that a PhD generates new knowledge and scientific discovery, whereas the DNP is more practice focused. Many DNP projects are listed on the website titled DNP Scholarly Projects: Archived and Searchable, which can be found at www.doctorsofnuringpractice.org.

THE NURSING PROCESS AND PROJECT MANAGEMENT

Although the concept of project management seems foreign to many, there is a common thread that applies it to the different types of work that nurses do. That thread is the nursing process, one of the first core principles of nursing practice nurses learn to use when delivering the best evidence-based patient care. The idea that nurses will understand and be able to apply the five basic principles of project management comes from its similarity to the five steps of the nursing process that are discussed in previous sections. The steps are similar to some project management terms and tasks; one just needs to learn the semantics between the nursing process and project management concepts. However, nurses, especially as they achieve more advanced levels of practice, will find many similarities between the processes of project management and the nursing process—the main difference being that they are working with a project instead of patients. These similarities are further explored in Chapter 2.

DEFINITION OF A PROJECT

A project is a planned set of interrelated tasks that need to be completed by certain dates. The specific beginning and ending dates indicate that one is engaged in a temporary process that may last weeks and/or months, but is not considered long term, such as the previous example of Amy planning her sister's wedding.

Many projects found in health care organizations have a specific or dedicated PM who designs, plans, and implements/builds and then applies the electronic health records (EHRs), based on the skills the PM has developed over previous projects or in graduate school. The PM needs to work with a team consisting of a variety of people, each with an area of expertise in the applications that will be built and applied in the system. For example, if the project were a clinical application for documentation, the build team would be separated into various smaller teams, such as a clinical documentation team composed primarily of nurses who had experience in documenting clinical notes. There would be a pharmacy team, medical team, and a list of other teams by department. These teams were brought together for the sole purpose of participating and assisting with the build of the system, and then would go back to their clinical jobs after the EHR has been installed. This process could take anywhere from 6 to 9 months to 1.5 years depending on the size of the installation. The project management processes and concepts described previously are very much like the nursing process discussed earlier and would represent some of the steps that Amy would need to understand for both her graduate practicum and her new role as manager.

WHAT IS PROJECT MANAGEMENT?

As discussed earlier, Amy told the CNO that she does not know what a project is, but was reassured that many tasks can take the form of a project, be they large or small, such as the practicum project or Amy's sister's wedding. They all require some sort of organization or framework and management to be successful.

Undertaking Project Management—Examples

For many, the idea of project management is daunting. The concept of being a PM is hard to comprehend, but actually taking on the role and being in charge is even more so. Understanding the basic concepts of project management, and how and where to apply them can be simple, regardless of the size or purpose of the project. As long as the basic project management concepts and organizational methods are understood and applied, it does not matter who takes on project management; the APN, DNP, CNO, or other health care professional, or those with other backgrounds such as nursing faculty. An APN may encounter any or all of these management philosophies on a project. Nursing faculty have to plan courses, set due dates, and essentially manage each course and task as if it were a small project. To summarize, project management is "undertaken to meet unique goals and objectives" (Nokes, 2007, p. 131) in a standardized way.

Constraints

PM and project management enthusiasts often discuss constraints. Constraints are limits, restrictions, and barriers to achieving the project goals and objectives. One of the most frequently discussed constraints is the ability to stay within the budget that was originally agreed to and most likely developed with consultation from the hospital's chief finance officer (CFO). Managing the budget, schedule, and resources—those hired to work on the project—are responsibilities of the PM, just as they would be for any type of task. Amy will learn how to manage these items in her management course as she first learns to develop what is called the "scope document." The scope document is developed out of the need for a documented plan that indicates when and how the plan will be carried out.

This type of plan also establishes boundaries of what will be done, how long it will take (time), how much it will cost, what resources/building supplies will be needed, and how many people it will take to get the work completed (resources). These three interdependencies—budget, schedule, and resources—are critical to a project's success and are discussed further during the design phase (Chapter 3). If one of these elements is out of plan, it will affect the other two; as will be discussed later.

PROJECT MANAGEMENT PROCESSES

Project management is a process of coordinating and directing team members to meet the formal, defined, approved goals and objectives outlined for the specific project. Managing a project will be accomplished using the skills developed in graduate school or on other projects while also managing the constraints discussed previously to stay on time and on budget as you monitor quality as well as team and stakeholder satisfaction and performance. This is best accomplished when using consistent, standard processes in an organized way to meet the project goals and objectives. As mentioned, the standard processes used in project management are very similar to the steps in the nursing process. They include a list of activities or tasks that need to be completed in each step before the next step can be started.

- Design (initiation)
- Plan
- Apply (implementation)
- Regulate or control; supervise (monitor)
- Conclude

While the overall project is being supervised, all steps must also be regulated or controlled. Although these five processes are the ones most frequently used, larger projects' processes may be broken into six or more components or phases so that the project can more easily be controlled. Organizing the project with specific steps adds a structure and a framework that is much easier to track and to change, if indicated.

PRINCIPLES OF PROJECT MANAGEMENT

Basic principles and an understanding of project management are frequently acquired over a number of projects; learning what works well and where to focus key time and resources takes time and experience. Just as with any project, including the wedding previously discussed or Amy's master's practicum project, some of the first questions to ask during a critical analysis are:

- Why are we doing this project?
- Why do we need it? Who will benefit?
- Does it fit the organization's strategic mission and plan?

The APN's role here is to help facilitate the discussions with end users who need the application in order to work effectively, information technologists, and other stakeholders. Additionally, if the APN has assumed the role of the PM, it will be important to fully understand the five project management processes and how to apply them as listed previously.

Not only is it critical that the APN in the role of PM be able to track, control, and closely monitor the five project management processes but to also understand other key responsibilities of project management, which are discussed in the following chapters. Those include regulating and controlling the project so that it is continually on time, on budget, and within scope of the project.

PROJECT MANAGEMENT: WHY DO WE NEED IT?

Historically, projects completed prior to 1950 were less organized and more haphazard than those undertaken today. According to Cleland and Gareis (2006), "It was in the 1950s, when project management was formally recognized as a distinct contribution arising from the management discipline" (pp. 1–4). Engineering was at the forefront of establishing project management. From the 1950s to today, the concept of project management has become a key management strategy in large corporations, such as IBM, Apple, Microsoft, other industries, and now, more recently, in health care where there is a need to put more formalized structure and organization to tasks carried out in organizations. Nurses use an organized approach when providing care to patients. Patient care management requires an organizational framework—organizing processes similar to those used in project management are used to manage patient care.

Driving Forces That Develop Skills

Initially recommended in the Institute of Medicine report (IOM, 2008) and with the advent of the American Recovery and Reinvestment Act (ARRA), which contained the Health Information Technology for Economic and Clinical Health Act (HITECH Act, 2009), came the mandate of what health care should do, including using EHRs to collect and monitor patient data, which further encouraged the use and development of technology by nurses, APNs, and other health care professionals. The Act's accompanying funding resources stimulated more rapid movement toward electronic data capture and health information exchanges (HIE; HealthIT.gov, n.d.). The HITECH Act is the portion of the ARRA that provides the U.S. Department of Health and Human Services (HHS) with the power to facilitate promotion and utilization of health information technology usage through government programs and Medicare and Medicaid, to levy fines if computer technology is not used in a meaningful way, and to collect and manage data in a way that will increase patient care efficiencies, improve care efficiencies, and cut health care dollars.

With the recommendations of the ARRA and accompanying mandates for hospitals to implement EHRs, there is an even greater need to implement standardized, organizing processes and methodologies to effectively and efficiently guide organizations through the many tasks needed to implement very complex EHRs in a very systematic way. Project management provides this standard process.

SUMMARY

This introductory chapter is designed to provide an overview for Amy, the new manager and MSN student, of some of the project management skills that an APN, DNP, CNO, or other health care professional needs when undertaking the design and implementation of a project. Chapter 2 discusses how well nurses and APNs fit into the PM role as it models many of the same concepts used in the nursing process.

The project management standards originally developed in the 1950s by engineers are explained. Although based on proven concepts, this text is focused on defining concepts in a way that non-project managers, such as APNs and others clinicians, will be better able to comprehend and apply to definitions and processes used on the business operations side of a health care organization.

REFERENCES

American Association of Colleges of Nursing (AACN). (2014). *Expanded roles for advanced practice nurses*. Retrieved from www.aacn.nche.edu

American Nurses Association (ANA). (2008). *Nursing informatics: Scope and standards of practice* (2nd ed.). Silver Spring, MD: Author.

American Nurses Association (ANA). (2010). *Nursing: Scope and standards of practice* (2nd ed.). Silver Spring, MD: Author.

American Recovery and Reinvestment Act (ARRA) Initiative, HITECH Act. (2009). HealthIT.gov. Retrieved from www.healthit.gov/policy-researchers-implementers/hitech-act

Association of College & Research Libraries. Retrieved from www.ala.org/ala/mgrps/divs/acrl/standards/standards

Cleland, D., & Gareis, R. (2006). *Global project management handbook* (pp. 1–4). New York, NY: McGraw-Hill Professional.

DNP scholarly projects: Archived and searchable. Retrieved from www.doctorsof nursingpractice.org

Institute of Medicine (IOM). (2008). *The future of nursing: Leading change, advancing health (National Academy of Sciences)*. Washington, DC: The National Academies Press.

Nokes, S. (2007). *The definitive guide to project management* (2nd ed., pp. 131–148). London, UK: Financial Times/Prentice-Hall.

CHAPTER 2

Advanced Practice Nurse Role Descriptions and Application of Project Management Concepts

LEARNING OBJECTIVES

Upon completion of this chapter, the reader will be able to:

1. Discuss the correlation between the nursing process and project management
2. List three roles that an advanced practice nurse (APN) can assume
3. Differentiate between information and computer literacy
4. Discuss the value of establishing a framework for a project
5. List two goals of using a standard process when designing a project

OUTLINE

- Key Terms
- History and Driving Forces to Develop Skills for the Role of the APN
- Correlation Between the Nursing Process and Project Management
- Understanding the Differences Between Information and Computer Literacy: Why Is This Important?
- APN and DNP Essential Skills
- Nurse Administrator Job Role and Essential Skills
- The Association of periOperative Registered Nurses' APN Job Description
- Competency Assessment

KEY TERMS

Competencies

Computer literacy

Doctor of nursing practice (DNP)

Health Information Technology
for Economic and Clinical
Health Act (HITECH)

Institute of Medicine (IOM)

Informatics nurse specialist (INS)

Information literacy

Nurse informaticist (NI)

Nursing process

The focus of this chapter is to help nurses understand the value and skills they will develop when learning the principles of project management that are very similar concepts to the nursing process, and are applied by an APN in practice. Not only are the steps that are used to manage patient care required in practice, nurses are expected to possess the skills and ability to apply concepts of project management in today's practice. The American Nurses Association (ANA; 2008) and the Healthcare Information Management Systems Society (HIMSS; 2014b) emphasize that "informatics competencies are needed by all nurses whether or not they specialize in informatics. As nurse settings become more ubiquitous computing environments, all nurses must be both information and computer literate (p. 1)." The methodology and technology used in informatics is part of project management in that the knowledge, techniques, and competencies required and developed using informatics help APNs to better manage their practice.

HISTORY AND DRIVING FORCES TO DEVELOP SKILLS FOR THE ROLE OF THE APN

A brief discussion of driving forces is provided in Chapter 1, but the major driving forces for nurses to advance their skills and practice levels are listed in the Institute of Medicine (IOM) report (2010): *The Future of Nursing: Leading Change, Advancing Health Through Better Data Collection and Improved Information Infrastructure.* This report sets forth a mandate and challenge to the practice of nursing; it suggests the need to transform the nursing profession as well as the health care system as a whole. In this significant report, there are eight core recommendations.

Of these, the ones most significant to nurses developing skills in project management are those listed here.

1. Expand opportunities for nurses to lead and diffuse collaborative improvement efforts
2. Ensure that nurses engage in lifelong learning, such as continuing toward a doctorate of nursing practice
3. Prepare and enable nurses to lead change to advance health
4. Build an infrastructure for the collection and analysis of interprofessional health care workforce data

Historically, in 2004 President George W. Bush outlined a plan to ensure that most Americans have an electronic health record (EHR) by 2014, and stated that "by computerizing health records we can avoid dangerous medical mistakes, reduce costs, and improve care" (President George W. Bush, State of the Union Address, January 20, 2004). Then in 2009, the Health Information Technology for Economic and Clinical Health (HITECH) Act, enacted as part of the American Recovery and Reinvestment Act of 2009, developed incentives for providers to become meaningful users of EHRs (American Recovery and Reinvestment ACT [ARRA] 2014). To be competent as an EHR user requires one to be competent in project management and informatics, specifically, data entry, analysis, facilitation between information technology (IT) and clinicians, workflow design, and change management (Health IT Policy, 2014).

This push to change the health care system, improve patient safety, and develop and implement EHRs has led to an increase in demand for project management skills as health systems realize that they need to update legacy systems in order to be more efficient when developing and managing a patient record. A critical point that was overlooked in all of these mandates was that very few in the workforce were competent or possessed the skills needed to implement any of the recommendations without extensive training. A report by the Health Resources and Services Administration (HRSA) suggests that the implementation of an EHR system requires skills in leadership and management of a project team (U.S. Department of Health and Human Services [HHS], 2014) that few possess. A partial list of additional project management skills needed to undertake any project, large or small, to keep it well organized and managed, also includes:

- Good communication skills and processes—both verbal and written
- Steps in the implementation process require close monitoring to stay on time and on budget

- Risk management; risks need to be defined, documented, tracked, and mitigated
- Monitoring resources
- Controlling quality

This list requires a skill mix of project management, computer literacy, and informatics. Finally, it should be noted that skills such as:

- Planning
- Organization
- Documentation of processes
- Assessment
- Change
- Reports and meetings

are needed in any management position or other leadership role, not just project management. Other roles and skills that APNs might assume are also discussed. Some of the information included was retrieved from job websites in a search for specific, updated roles and skills required today.

In the past, the leaders and committees that mandated the driving forces identified the tasks and skills needed to move health care reform forward. But many times when organizations tried to hire someone with the skills needed for the job, such as managing an EHR implementation, they found a gap in both the skill levels and education of APNs with regard to management skills. APNs are proficient in assessing and providing patient care but lack the management skills needed to plan and organize a clinic, manage resources, budgets, time, and many other aspects of project management.

CORRELATION BETWEEN THE NURSING PROCESS AND PROJECT MANAGEMENT

Although the concept of project management seems foreign to many, there is a common thread that applies to the different types of work that nurses do (i.e., the nursing process—one of the first core principles of nursing practice that nurses learn to use when delivering the best evidence-based patient care). The suggestion that nurses will understand and be able to apply the five basic principles of project management arises from project management's similarity to the five steps of the nursing process. The steps and phases are similar to some project management terms and tasks, but differences may be only an issue of semantics. Ultimately, nurses, especially as they achieve more advanced levels in their practice, will find many similarities between the processes of project management and the nursing process. The main difference is that they are working with a project instead of patients (Table 2.1).

In summary, just as the nursing process provides an organizing framework for patient care management, the project management processes provide the organizational framework for a project or other roles where an organizing framework would be useful (Figures 2.1 and 2.2).

TABLE 2.1
Correlation of the Nursing Process to Project Management Concepts

Nursing Process	Project Management
1. Assessment—collect and analyze patient data	1. Design/Initiate project—current state workflow analysis; gap analysis
2. Diagnosis; develop pre-care plan	2. Develop project plan
3. Outcomes plan; goal development	3. Implement project plan
4. Implement care plan	4. Monitor and control project
5. Evaluate plan; update plan	5. Close project; evaluate lessons learned

Sipes (2014).

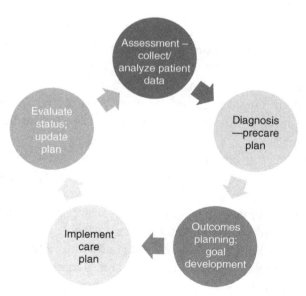

FIGURE 2.1 The Five Steps of the Nursing Process

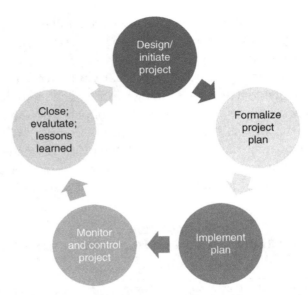

FIGURE 2.2 The Five Phases of Project Management
From Sipes (2014).

UNDERSTANDING THE DIFFERENCES BETWEEN INFORMATION AND COMPUTER LITERACY: WHY IS THIS IMPORTANT?

As APNs develop more advanced leadership and management skills, they must also become more information and computer literate. As noted earlier, the ANA statement emphasizes that "informatics competencies are needed by all nurses whether or not they specialize in informatics. As nurse settings become more ubiquitous computing environments, all nurses must be both information and computer literate" (ANA, 2008, p. 2).

It is important to understand the differences between information and computer literacy because they are required today as part of demonstrated competency in information management, which includes applying the concepts and framework of project management. There are several definitions of computer literacy. A basic definition is as follows: Computer literacy is the knowledge and ability to use computers and related technology efficiently, understand computer concepts and limitations, and possess a range of skills covering levels from elementary use to programming and advanced problem solving.

In addition to computer literacy, understanding the concepts of information literacy is essential to developing skills needed by the APN, especially as nursing today is becoming more high-tech.

> The beginning of the 21st century has been called the Information Age because of the explosion of information output and information sources. Information literacy forms the basis for lifelong learning. It is common to all disciplines, to all learning environments, and to all levels of education. It enables learners to master content and extend their investigations, become more self-directed, and assume greater control over their own learning. Information literacy is the set of skills needed to understand, find, retrieve, analyze, and use information. (Association of College & Research Libraries, 2014, p. 1)

"Computer literacy is a core competency needed in health care, and should be taught in nursing curricula at all levels. In addition, information literacy must be integrated into practice and used to support knowledge management. These are the foundations of informatics competencies" (ANA, 2010, p. 5). To be considered literate in computers an APN should have experience and competencies when using computers and applications as well as understand some of the basic techniques needed in order to support other nurses and peers. Again, as mentioned earlier, the APN employs principles of both informatics and project management to be considered competent and literate in computers and information technology (IT). As indicated, many comparisons have been made between the five steps of the nursing process and project management. As noted by Research Gate (2014), nurses are well suited for IT implementations, which follows the nursing process of assessment, diagnosis, planning, implementation, and evaluation.

The American Association of Colleges of Nursing (AACN, 2006, 2011) defined essential and expected competencies for nursing informatics education and graduation that apply to developing project management skills. The competencies expected for graduation are defined at three levels: those required for bachelor's of science in nursing (BSN), master's of science in nursing (MSN), and doctorate of nursing practice (DNP). For example, competencies expected at the DNP level for graduation include the ability to design, select, evaluate, and use processes; to analyze and communicate critical elements; to develop and execute plans; and to demonstrate leadership. All of these competencies are the same as those expected from a project manager (PM).

"Informatics and electronic health/medical records are being mandated by Federal mandates with professional organizations encouraging the adoption of such electronic records in clinical practice. Health information record systems are now functional systems through which nurses navigate technology, documents, and plan patient care" (Gardner & Jones, 2012, p. 1702). Because of the rapidly evolving changes in health information requirements and technology, there is also a need for nurses to acquire higher level computer and information competencies.

The role of the PM is critical to the success of a project. Many times leadership may overlook the value of a PM with the notion that another person in a leadership role can also assume the role while also completing his or her other duties. It is important to note that the role of the PM is different and should be different from operations or other functional managers. The role of the APN as a seasoned PM will bring skills and knowledge to the project, including a thorough understanding of the key concepts and principles of project management.

APN AND DNP ESSENTIAL SKILLS

This book defines the functional areas and competencies as well as the accountabilities and activities required in the role of a PM. Although this book will primarily be used as a course text, resource, and guide, the basic concepts and processes in the book will help develop and guide skills needed for other health informatics specialties and other health care providers who may be assuming a project management role in the health care industry or who need to have organizing guidelines necessary to develop a project for a graduate practicum in a master's or doctoral program.

According to the ANA, the following competencies are essential for all beginning nurses:

- Basic computer literacy, including the ability to use basic desktop applications and electronic communication
- The ability to use IT to support clinical and administrative processes, which presumes information literacy to support evidence-based practice

- The ability to access data and perform documentation via computerized patient records
- The ability to support patient safety initiatives via the use of IT (ANA, 2008)

But many nurses, even at the advanced level, do not have the basic competencies needed for most nursing jobs today. More than ever, nursing is considered a high-tech discipline. For nurses entering an APN program, especially in graduate school, the project management framework is beneficial in courses where the goal of the course is to assess, develop, and implement best practices for a project that might address a specific practice issue for a health care organization. This is especially important when collaborating with others in nursing practice, nursing leadership, or other fields of study or health care disciplines. Most nurses who enter into graduate school are unfamiliar with project management processes until they realize its correlation to the nursing process that they have used for years. As they continue the career path through graduate school, they will develop and apply the organizational skills they have learned, but now it will be while designing and planning the framework they will use to develop a practicum project required for graduation.

Additionally, at this point in the graduate program, the APN will need to evaluate his or her competencies of basic computer skills as well as the information and computer literacy described here. These skills will have to be assessed prior to taking on the role of a PM, as they are a basic requirement to function well in that role.

NURSE ADMINISTRATOR JOB ROLE AND ESSENTIAL SKILLS

The ANA and American Nurses Credentialing Center (ANCC) education requirements and skills outline core abilities necessary for the nurse administrator. These include:

- Ability and experience to use management skills
- Ability to embrace change and innovations to manage resource effectively
- Ability to negotiate and resolve conflict
- Ability to communicate effectively

The nurse administrator is a "registered nurse whose primary responsibility is to manage health care delivery services … in a variety of settings … and must be prepared … in such fields as information management and evidence-based care and management" (ANA, 2014, p. 6). As a nurse executive, one must develop and implement evaluation of six standards for nurse administrators and executives, including assessment, diagnosis of problems, identification of outcomes, planning, implementation, and evaluation as well as other organizational responsibilities. Evidence-based management is an important process that should be implemented in health care because the work environment in health care experiences greater turbulence, chaos, and instability than it does in other disciplines. Untested and dated management practices are no longer useful and may even be detrimental to patient care. Roles that use this process are listed in the following text, although the specific content within a project will depend on the specialty area; however, the basic principles and processes are the same for any project that might be developed.

THE ASSOCIATION OF PERIOPERATIVE REGISTERED NURSES' APN JOB DESCRIPTION

The Association of periOperative Registered Nurses (AORN) defines an APN as a nurse practitioner (NP), clinical nurse specialist (CNS), certified registered nurse anesthetist (CRNA), or certified nurse-midwife (CNM). Some of the job functions and skills necessary for an APN per the AORN are that the APN should be able to:

- Direct patient care
- Provide consultation for nursing staff by implementing improvements in health care delivery systems
- Assess, plan, implement, evaluate, and document care (project management skills)

The manager roles require that the APN be experienced in staffing, budgeting, and resource management—all project management skills.

- Manage staff, such as certified nursing assistants, registered nurses, licensed practical nurses, surgical technologists, and

other allied health care providers; schedule staff; hire and fire staff; mentor staff (resource management)
- Maintain department or unit's budget (budgeting)
- Communicate organizational issues to the staff (communication)
- Oversee daily activities within their department or unit (project management)
- Collaborate with other departments and physicians on departmental issues

At the director level, AORN requires that the APN skills include, but are not limited to, responsibility for the operation of the department and for the measurement, assessment, and continuous improvement of the department's performance.

The Nurse Practitioner and Clinical Nurse Specialist

NPs and CNSs prepared at the master's or doctoral level perform advanced practice nursing in an assigned specialty population throughout the continuum of care. The CNS serves in all three spheres of influence: complex patient care and research, systems processes and policies, and staff development and nursing practice. The CNS influences patient- and family-centered care and evidence-based nursing practice, promotes best practices for the interprofessional patient care team, and promotes evidence-based organizational change to meet the needs of the assigned population. This CNS is responsible for the development, implementation, promotion, and day-to-day coordination of this program. Skills also include leading groups and implementing change, as well as the ability to respond and manage change. The CNS must have the ability to communicate effectively both orally and in writing, manage multiple simultaneous tasks and prioritize appropriately, as well as have knowledge of dynamics of group process (Clinical Nurse Specialist Jobs, 2014).

Many times, NPs and CNSs manage and own their own practices. They also achieve a higher level of education, the DNP.

The Nurse Informaticist

The nurse informaticist (NI) differentiates from other informatics specialties, such as medicine, pharmacy, and dentistry, where the focus is more on database management. Each informatics specialty is aligned uniquely with its primary role, requiring that informatics nurse specialists (INSs) augment their base of nursing knowledge with unique informatics skills. In the past, the definition of the NI focused solely on data collection and the use of data; many organizations still are not choosing to implement the use of an NI until post–electronic medical record (EMR) implementation (when electronic data are robust). According to the ANA, in 2008, the beginning nurse focused primarily on developing and using skills that rely on the ability to retrieve and enter data in an electronic format that is relevant to patient care, the analysis and interpretation of information as part of planning care, the use of informatics applications designed for nursing practice, and the implementation of policies relevant to information (ANA, 2008, p. 1). According to the HIMSS (2014a) statement regarding NI functions, the NI has advanced from a discipline previously focused on EMR implementation to one that ultimately facilitates and optimizes technology and informatics tools that help clinicians provide better care and positive health outcomes for patients as they monitor the outcomes. Additionally, it is important to note that the NI role is rapidly evolving in the functional areas and now plays a more integral role in the early planning phases of system development and management. This is why the NI and INS need to develop project management skills.

The Informatics Nurse Specialist

The INS is often responsible for implementing or coordinating projects involving multiple disciplines. The INS is expected to interact with professionals involved in all phases of the information systems' life cycle and with professionals in all aspects of system utilization. "Both the INS and NI support consumers, patients, nurses, and other providers in their decision making in all roles and settings. This support is accomplished through the use of information structures, information process and information technology" (ANA, 2008, p. 1). ANA (2008) defines the level 3 nurse as an INS who is a registered nurse with advanced preparation and knowledge in information management.

A partial list of skills include the ability to incorporate critical thinking, process skills, data management skills, project management and systems development lifecycle skills, and computer skills into areas of nursing practice. Some of the more advanced competencies that the INS will have include:

- Proficiency with informatics applications to support all areas of nursing practice, including project management, quality-improvement activities, research, as well as system design, development, analysis, implementation, support, maintenance, and evaluation—all skills that a PM possesses
- Fiscal management
- Skills in critical thinking, data management and processing, decision making, system development, and computer skills
- Identification and provision of data for decision making (ANA, 2008)

An INS in the role of administrator and leader would potentially work as a chief nursing information officer (CNIO) (HIMSS, 2014a, p. 4). In a midlevel management role, the INS's activities might include conducting "a needs analysis, design, development, evaluation, and implementation" of a system (ANA, 2008, p. 18). This is an area that would require project management skills.

Chief Nursing Information Officer

If the APN were to assume a job as a CNIO, the skills and expectations would include (per the HIMSS website's job description) the ability to:

- Lead the region in the strategy, development, and implementation of IT to support nursing, nursing practice, and clinical applications, by collaborating with area chief nursing officers (CNOs) on the clinical and administrative decision-making process
- Develop clinical systems strategy by collaborating with the regional chief medical information officer (CMIO)
- Optimize the use of existing clinical systems for nurses, physicians, and other multidisciplinary care providers by attending to their information management needs

- Practice an executive nature, comprised of complex leadership and administrative components, associated with critical health care issues and activities that influence the organizational mission, health care, and policy
- Collaborate with other executives for strategic planning, decision making, and problem solving, as well as developing resource utilization strategies to improve organizational performance
- Use project management experience to advance projects (HIMSS, 2014a)

Doctorate of Nursing Practice

The doctorate of nursing practice (DNP) graduate's practice includes not only direct care but also a focus on the needs of patients, a target population, a set of populations, or a broad community. The DNP

- Must be able to conceptualize new care delivery models that are based in contemporary nursing science and that are feasible within current organizational, political, cultural, and economic perspectives
- Must be skilled in working within organizational and policy arenas and in the actual provision of patient care alone and/or with others
- Must understand principles of practice management, including conceptual and practical strategies for balancing productivity with quality of care
- Must be able to assess the impact of practice policies and procedures on meeting the health needs of the patient populations with whom he or she practices
- Must be proficient in quality-improvement strategies and in creating and sustaining changes at the organizational and policy levels
- Must be able to manage corresponding change management in organizational arrangements, manage organizational and professional cultures, and manage the financial structures necessary to support practice
- Must be able to evaluate the cost-effectiveness of care and use principles of economics and finance to redesign effective and realistic care delivery strategies

- Must be able to organize care to address emerging practice problems and the ethical dilemmas that emerge as new diagnostic and therapeutic technologies evolve
- Must be able to assess risk and collaborate with others to manage risks ethically, based on professional standards
- Must be able to design, select, and use information systems/technology to evaluate programs of care, outcomes of care, and care systems; using information systems/technology the DNP must be able to apply budget and productivity tools, practice information systems and decision supports, and use web-based learning or intervention tools to support decision making and manage and provide leadership

To summarize, skills needed by any or all of the roles defined include:

- Organization skills, management skills
- Clinical reengineering—workflow and gap analysis
- Change management
- Work processes support
- Information management
- Time management
- Resource management
- Leadership
- Communication skills
- Strategic planning
- Decision making and decision support
- Problem solving
- Budget development and cost monitoring

All of the skills listed, and others, are required of a PM. During the initial design and planning phase of the project, the APN will be expected to have skill and experience in developing the management and budget tools that will be needed to track the various project functions.

Further, because roles are frequently confused with position titles and with the lack of standardization in the new specialty of nursing informatics, the ANA has provided a description of some of the functional areas for INSs and NIs that are still relevant and are evolving today. These include:

- Administration, leadership, and management
- Analysis

- Compliance and integrity management
- Consultation
- Coordination, facilitation, and integration
- Development
- Educational and professional development
- Policy development and advocacy
- Research and evaluation (ANA, 2008, pp. 17–18)

The expanded use of health information technology (HIT) promotes interprofessional development and collaboration, as well as patient involvement in the utilization of health care devices. This will require the APN to address all environments and all levels of user ability to accommodate the various devices being developed (Table 2.2).

Although the survey referred to in Table 2.3 was completed by HIMSS for NIs, the directive for all nurses to have skills in project management has been recognized and recommended by such organizations as ANA, ANCC, and the Quality and Safety Education

TABLE 2.2
Partial List of Essential Roles and Skills of an APN

As change agents	An inherent function of the APN is that of a change agent, involving collaboration and consultation with other health care providers (AACN)
As leaders	Have excellent communication skills, conduct risk assessment, coalition building with business acumen, and have strategic application knowledge
Are comfortable with change and complexity in dynamic environments	The use of evidence-based practice necessitates the implementation of change; the APN as change agent (Medscape, 2014)
Able to guide and cultivate people skills	Guides others in the development of effective oral and written communication skills, including communication with project stakeholders (www .healthsystem.virginia.edu)
Have a broad and flexible toolkit of techniques	Adapt his or her approach to the context and constraints of each project, knowing that no "one size" can fit all the variety of projects
Have the knowledge to develop and utilize a variety of tools	Utilize the tools to track the project progress from start to completion
Take ownership for the project	Assume responsibility and accountability for the project

APN, advanced practice nurse.
Adapted from the AACN (2008, p. 18).

TABLE 2.3
HIMSS NI Workforce Survey Top Five Job
Responsibilities—Application to APNs

#1 Systems implementation

#2 Systems development

#3 Quality initiatives

#4 Liaison with IT, other clinicians

#5 Strategic planning

HIMSS, Healthcare Information and Management Systems Society; IT, information technology; NI, nurse informaticist.
Data from HIMSS (2011).

for Nurses (QSEN) survey funded by the Robert Wood Johnson Foundation (RWJF). The table lists results from the NI workforce survey of the top five job responsibilities. This survey was conducted by the HIMSS in 2011. The emphasis on collecting this data was to demonstrate that the NIs and INSs should be employed earlier than later with an EHR system implementation. This survey provides evidence that NIs and INSs should not only be employed after the fact for data collection but during the first decision-making processes.

COMPETENCY ASSESSMENT

Today many colleges, universities, and national organizations require that all nurses complete a competency assessment that provides feedback regarding the level of skills the nurse has and the skills needed in order to achieve a particular skill level. Today, employers rely more heavily on national organizations and universities to provide the necessary education and certifications the nurse will need for a specific job.

SUMMARY

The purpose of this chapter is to provide some of the nursing roles the APN can assume today, if he or she has the skills needed to meet expectations identified in the job descriptions. It also provides an overview, including a partial list of role expectations needed as a PM. The following chapters provide the knowledge, tools, and recommendations on how to acquire and develop the skills needed to assume the role of PM or apply a framework needed to complete a practicum in graduate school courses. It will provide opportunities to practice using the tools, methodology, and processes inherent in each phase of the project—from designing, planning, implementing, monitoring, and controlling the project and, finally, closing the project and conducting an evaluation of the process or lessons learned. Today's workforce is expected to possess higher level knowledge and skills in order to be competent and competitive in the job market.

REFERENCES

American Association of Colleges of Nursing. (2008). *The Essentials of Master's Education in Nursing.* Retrieved from http://www.aacn.nche.edu/education-resources/BaccEssentials08.pdf

American Nurses Association (ANA). (2008). *Nursing informatics: Scope and standards of practice.* Silver Spring, MD: Nursesbooks.org

American Nurses Association (ANA). (2009). *Nursing administration: scope and standards of practice.* Silver Spring, MD: Nursesbooks.org

American Nurses Association (ANA). (2010). *Nursing: Scope and standards of practice* (2nd ed.). Silver Spring, MD: Nursesbooks.org

American Nurses Credentialing Center (ANCC). www.nursecredentialing.org

American Recovery and Reinvestment Act (ARRA) Initiative. (2014). *HITECH Act.* Retrieved from www.healthit.gov/policy-researchers-implementers/hitech-act

Association of College & Research Libraries. (2014). *Advancing learning, transforming scholarship: What is computer literacy?* Retrieved from www.ala.org/acrl/issues

Clinical Informatics RSS Feed. (2014). Retrieved from www.himss.org/ASP/himssNewsRSS.asp

Clinical Nurse Specialist Jobs. (2014). Retrieved from www.jobs2/view.com

Gardner, C., & Jones, S. (2012, June). Utilization of academic electronic medical records in undergraduate nursing education. *Online Journal of Nursing Informatics (OJNI)*, 16(2). Available at http://ojni.org/issues/?p=1702

Healthcare Information and Management Systems Society (HIMSS). (2007). *2007 HIMSS nursing informatics survey.* Retrieved from www.himss.org/content/files/surveyresults/2007NursingInformatics

Healthcare Information and Management Systems Society (HIMSS). (2014a). *Chief nursing information officer (CNIO) job descriptions.* Retrieved from www.himss.org/files/File

Healthcare Information and Management Systems Society (HIMSS). (2014b). *Informatics competencies: Integration into practice.* Retrieved from http://himss.files.cms-plus.com/2014Conference

Health IT Policy. (2014). *Implementation of EHRs; meaningful use.* Retrieved from http://healthit.gov/policy-researchers-implementers/health-it-legislation

Institute of Medicine (IOM). (2010). *The future of nursing: Leading change, advancing health, better data collection and improved information infrastructure.* Washington, DC: The National Academies Press.

Institute of Medicine (IOM). (2012). *Health IT and patient safety: Building safer systems for better care.* Washington, DC: The National Academies Press.

Medscape. (2014). *Role of the advanced practice nurse.* Retrieved from www.medscape.com

NI Toolbox & NI Knowledge Repository. (2014). www.himss.org/ni

President George W. Bush, State of the Union Address. (2004, January 20). *Transforming health care: The president's health information technology plan.* Retrieved from http://georgewbush whitehouse.archives.gov

Project Management Institute. (2013). *A guide to the project management body of knowledge (PMBOK® Guide)* (5th ed., p. 5). Author.

Research Gate. (2014). *Is project management essential for charge nurses, head nurses, nursing supervisors, and in other managerial nursing positions?* Retrieved February 21, 2014, from www.researchgate.net

U.S. Department of Health and Human Services. (2014). *What skills are needed to implement and support an EHR system?* Retrieved from www.hrsa.gov/healthit/toolbox

Zaccagnini, M., & White, K., (2011). *The doctor of nursing practice essentials: A new model for advanced practice nursing.* Sudbury, MA: Jones & Bartlett.

Phases of Project Management

CHAPTER 3

Design/Initiation: Project Management—Phase 1

LEARNING OBJECTIVES

Upon completion of this chapter, the reader will be able to:

1. Define *charter*
2. Define *scope*
3. Describe three topics defined in a charter
4. Describe two tasks found in a scope document
5. List two items that need to be included in a measurable objective

OUTLINE

- Key Terms
- Gap Analysis
- Project Goals and Objectives
- Project Charter
- Scope and Scope Creep
- Statement of Work Criteria
- Project Timeline
- Organizational Structures—Pros and Cons
- Team Selection and Formation
- PM Roles and Responsibilities

KEY TERMS

Charter	Matrix organization
Current state	Scope
Design/initiation phase	SMART objectives
Functional organization	Stakeholder analysis
Gap analysis	Statement of work (SOW)
Goals	Timeline

The role of the project manager (PM) is critical to the success of a project. Many times leadership may overlook the value of a PM, with the belief that another person in a leadership role can also assume the PM role while also completing his or her other duties. It is important to note that the role of the PM is and should be different from operations of other functional managers. "Each functional manager is responsible for a particular division, section or project. The functional manager is usually selected for his technical expertise and ability to control the day-to-day operations of the division" (Benjamin, n.d.). As a seasoned PM, the advanced practice nurse (APN) will bring skills and knowledge to the project, including a thorough understanding of the key concepts and principles of project management as well as the various skills possessed by an advance practice clinician; combining these skill sets enables the APN PM to facilitate and tie the two together.

Chapter 3 provides an overview of the different steps in a project. The first of the five phases of a project is the design or initiation phase. The initiation process starts when it has been determined that a new project or update to an existing project is needed. The initiation phase includes conducting all the activities necessary to begin formally planning the project, which is the second step or phase. The initiation phase typically begins with the assignment of the PM, hiring the project team, and ends when the project team has the information needed to begin developing a detailed plan and budget. At which point the project team moves to phase 2—planning, which is discussed in Chapter 4.

Activities required during the design/initiation phase include identification of the project sponsor, and developing the scope and charter documents that, when signed off, formally authorize the project. This is the phase during which the initial timeline for the project is developed, when the need for the project is clearly justified and defined, and measurable project objectives are developed.

Depending on the project, if part of an ongoing organizational implementation of an electronic medical records (EMRs) system, the initiation phase will include a review of past lessons learned. This is also the phase during which the stakeholders will need to be defined. The stakeholders are those who have an interest in the project, such as end users, project sponsors, and project team members, to name a few. At this point it will be important to request representatives for end users as there may be many—such as staff nurses—who may have differing ideas of what should be accomplished with the project. The stakeholders will define what the project should accomplish, such as the deliverables or end results of the project. They will also help define the assumptions, critical success factors (CSF), timeline, and resources. High-level stakeholders, such as a vice president, "C" levels (chief executive officer [CEO], chief informatics officer (CIO), chief nursing informatics officer [CNIO], and chief financial officer [CFO]), or other leadership, will help define the project budget.

It will be important to understand the organizational philosophy for project management, whether it has a methodology, and what the PM role will be, including levels of authority and accountability. All of these tasks need to be clearly defined and then entered into project management documents during the planning phase, prior to the kick-off meeting that formally launches the project.

GAP ANALYSIS

Current State

The first step when launching any project is to conduct and analyze the "current state." Current state refers to reviewing the "what is"—what is currently happening—and then look to define what and/or where the gaps might be—what is missing or what could make it better. For example, one of the reasons a project might have been proposed is the need for a remodel, an upgrade, to solve some problem, such as long patient wait times, or to add something new that would expedite a process. Overall, the project is being implemented to meet a need, and the need or gap should be justified with documentation of workflows to show the gaps.

When beginning to diagram a workflow, the first step is to start by drawing boxes that will represent each step in the process until arriving at a step where there is a gap in the flow—the gap analysis (see Figure 3.1)—the gaps in the process should be clearly evident. It is important to do this first by just sketching the diagram quickly on a note pad while working with others who may be providing information so that thought processes are not lost. As frequently happens, the process will include a review and may be revised a number of times. As end users start to think through the processes, with repeated review they will begin to remember more details, especially if they are working with others to document the workflow. After several iterations have been completed, the diagram can be formally documented, especially if using a program called Microsoft Visio. If one is not familiar with this program, there may be a steep learning curve to learn how to use it, but there may be no time to do so. Many times organizations have someone on the project who has experience using the application.

Documentation of the gap analysis is conducted to define what parts of the workflow process are not working well, which are taking too much time, such as redundant charting, or other steps in a process that may cause extra work. This process review may be able to identify a missing application that will greatly speed up a process or function.

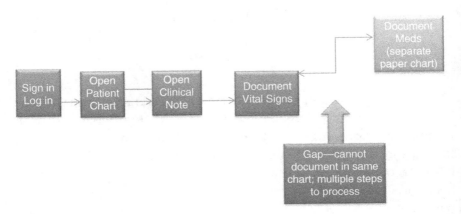

FIGURE 3.1 Current State Electronic Clinical Documentation With Gap in Charting
From Sipes (2014).

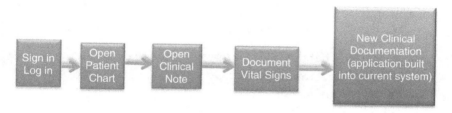

FIGURE 3.2 Future State Electronic Clinical Documentation: Gap Resolved
From Sipes (2014).

Future State

The next step is to design the "future state" application. There are many considerations when implementing the future state or "what will be," such as the impact and change the new process will cause the entire organization. Change can be very difficult; most people do not like change and are content with status quo. Change management techniques and plan as well as tool development are discussed in Chapters 4 and 5. The future state diagrams will show the new changes in workflow and where the proposed changes will occur (see Figure 3.2).

PROJECT GOALS AND OBJECTIVES

Critical to the detail in this document is the inclusion of measurable, well-defined goals and objectives. A goal is defined as a general statement about some task or project that needs to be accomplished. The objectives define the steps that determine how the goal(s) will be accomplished and help keep the project moving. Many PMs who create management documents find it difficult to develop well-defined, specific goals and objectives, only to discover later that they were missing a task, due date, or owner of a specific task, and therefore cannot adequately track whether this missing item has been completed. Well-defined goals and objectives will include details and metrics, such as:

- Number of units
- Specific tasks to be completed
- Due dates
- Owner/responsibility

You can think of a well-defined objective by answering the five "W" questions of who, what, where, when, and why and an "H," how.

- Who and what department or role needs to do the activities?
- Who will the project impact?
- Who will pay for the project?
- Who is making the decisions?
- What are the benefits and to whom?
- Where will this occur?
- When will the different activities be completed?
- Why is this project being done?
- How will this be completed—list of tasks, resources? (Sipes, 2014)

Writing SMART Objectives

The objectives should be developed as SMART objectives, meaning they need to be specific, measurable, achievable (attainable), relevant, and timely (Table 3.1).

The key to developing critical measurable objectives is having collectable data that is adequate for measuring change (Issel, 2004).

PROJECT CHARTER

What Is a Charter?

In this phase of design a number of key project management documents are created, including the charter, which adds the framework for the who, what, when, why, where, and how so the project can proceed, including the formal sign-off by key leadership and stakeholders, which authorizes the project and gives authority to the PM. A needs assessment, also referred to as the workflow gap analysis, includes a review of the current state of the project as well as anticipated future state information. The workflow analysis helps to define and organize basic draft ideas into a more comprehensive format that is easier to follow. The needs assessment contains the

TABLE 3.1
Goal and SMART Objectives

Goal	Implement Staff Training Project for Nursing Department
Objectives: ■ S = Specific; answer the five "W" questions	■ The training for the clinical documentation application in the EHR will be implemented for 5N Med–Surg Nursing ■ Training will start March 15, 2014, by staff super-user trainers prior to the system going live
■ M = Measurable; how will you know when you have accomplished the objective?	■ The education will be accomplished when 35 RN staff from 5N Med–Surg Nursing completes the training ■ They will need to pass the competency test with 85% within 2 weeks of completing the training that starts on March 15, 2014, ending on March 30, 2014
■ A = Achievable; will you be able to achieve it within the triple constraints—time, budget, resources?	■ The time allotted to complete the training was approved by leadership on February 1 ■ The budget to complete the training was approved by leadership on February 1 ■ Three additional trainers have been hired and completed their training on March 1
■ R = Relevant; do the objectives comply with the organization's mission?	■ The objectives comply with the organization's mission goals of implementing an EHR in NM Health Systems in 2014, to improve patient safety and access to health care
■ T = Timely; do you have due dates for every task?	■ Metrics for each objective are included, e.g., number of staff, number of trainers, location, and due dates

EHR, electronic health record.
From Sipes (2014). Adapted from Writing SMART Objectives (2009). cdc.gov.

evaluation of the business need for the project as well as the antici-pated outcome of the project.

The project charter is based on the outcomes of the gap analysis; it also defines costs, lists tasks in the form of a schedule, and contains a Gantt chart and the deliverables. To develop a project charter you will need to identify the information found in Table 3.2.

TABLE 3.2
Project Charter Content

Project Charter

Title of project:

Objective of project:

Background/justification:

Scope statement summary:

Project participants:

Executive Steering Team (EST)

Name	Title	Department

Roles and responsibilities:

Time requirement:

Total estimated hours per member:

Project Steering Team (PST)

Name	Title	Department

Roles and responsibilities:

Time requirement:

Total estimated hours per member:

Project Work Team

Name	Title	Department

Project governance

Roles and responsibilities:

Time requirement:

Total estimated hours per member:

Other resources: (vendors; administrative, clinical, technical resources that will be required)

Activities: (will be listed in project plan)

Deliverables: (to support scope document)

Time frame:

Special considerations: (assumptions, constraints, directives from management)

Approval and sign-off: (project sponsor agrees with scope of activities and deliverables)

Name	Title	Department

Sipes (2014).

SCOPE AND SCOPE CREEP

The scope document is a formal document that details how the project will be managed and what the project requirements are. It defines the boundaries of what can and cannot be done. After the scope document is approved by the key stakeholders, any additional or further change will need to go through the change management process (described in Chapters 4 and 5) and be approved by stakeholders and other key leadership. The scope document should address the problem or opportunity that will be resolved with the implementation of the project. It defines the project goal and objectives and the metrics that will be used to determine the success of the project. When the scope document is completed it will need to be included as one document with the charter.

Mitigating Scope Creep

Unapproved change in scope—known as scope creep—can cause delays in the project and/or budget overruns, especially if there are issues such as acquiring additional human and other resources such as equipment. Scope creep occurs when something is forgotten and not included in the original requirements document but must be itemized. The two major components that need to be evaluated in scope creep are:

- Defining the extent of the project change
- Completing an assessment of the impact of the change on the organization

To determine how changes will impact the project, different attributes will need to be analyzed and documented. Those include, but are not limited to:

- The type of impact the change will have
- Impact on project schedule and timeline
- Whether the project can incorporate and accommodate the change
- What will happen to the project if the change is not implemented
- How manageable the change is—time, cost, resources, quality

TABLE 3.3
Scope Statement

Organization's name:	
Project's name:	
Scope document:	
Project manager:	Priority level:
Sponsors:	
Mission statement:	
Measurable project objectives:	
Justification:	
Implementation strategy:	
Project resources:	
Completion date:	
Measures of success:	
Assumptions:	
Constraints:	

Approvals

	Signatures:	Date:
Manager and sponsor:		
Project manager approval:		
Owner approval:		

Sipes (2014).

The CSF will also need to be defined, including a timeline for completion of all deliverables. Content that will need to be included in the scope statement is listed in Table 3.3.

Difference Between Charter and Scope—Getting Approval

A project charter defines the purpose of the project and includes the measurable objectives (see Table 3.1). It also includes a list of the high-level requirements for the project as well as the project description. It should include expected milestones and a budget. It includes the PM's job description, with the roles and responsibility definitions, and clearly defines the authority levels, including reporting structure. Finally, it lists who the authorizing person(s) is and includes requirements for how different aspects of the project will be approved.

TABLE 3.4
Key Differences Between Charter and Scope Statement

Project Scope	Project Charter
▪ Describes project	▪ Defines purpose and description of the project
▪ Specifies project deliverables	▪ Outlines measurable objectives and expected milestones
▪ Specifies what is in scope and what is not included	▪ Defines high-level requirements
▪ Defines the user acceptance criteria	▪ Lists approval requirements; sign-off authorizes project
▪ Lists constraints	▪ Defines project manager roles and responsibilities and the reporting structure
▪ Lists assumptions	▪ Contains the budget

Adapted from Banner (2014).

In contrast, the scope document includes a description of the project and defines the project deliverables. It defines what is in scope and what is not included in the scope of the project. It also defines the user acceptance criteria, and includes constraints and assumptions for the project (Table 3.4).

STATEMENT OF WORK CRITERIA

If the organization or project requires a statement of work (SOW) it can be one of the most important things that you might need to develop in place of the project charter and scope documents. However, many of the other documents you will develop as a PM would be redundant if you are also required to create and include a SOW. This informational note is only included here as some organizations do require all documents, especially government organizations. A SOW will include:

- Background, requirements, and history of proposed project
- Charter documents
- Scope document

- Objectives of the project
- Tasks to be completed in the project
- Project schedule
- Project milestones
- Deliverables of the project
- Resource management and budget

The SOW will include the documented five "W"s and an "H"—who, what, where, why, when, and how (Sipes, 2014). The SOW is a legal contract between a number of contractors, the organization, and leadership. Some organizations require that you also include the assumptions found in the scope. When this document is completed, it will need to be reviewed by legal and leadership for approval and sign-off as approval for the project to proceed.

PROJECT TIMELINE

The project timeline is another extremely important document that must be developed at the outset of a project. This document provides a quick view of the overall project and includes high-level milestones to be completed each week or month, depending on the length of the project. This document should be reviewed at every weekly project and stakeholder meeting to validate the project is on track.

Many organizations keep a large wall map of a timeline, such as the timeline shown in Figure 3.3, as a constant reminder of where the project is and where it is going. Frequently, the timeline includes detail to keep team members and others who are involved in the project informed; it is a key to good communication.

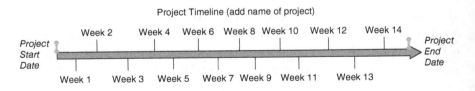

FIGURE 3.3 Project Timeline
From Sipes (2014).

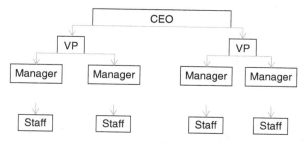

FIGURE 3.4 Functional Organization
From Sipes (2014).

ORGANIZATIONAL STRUCTURES— PROS AND CONS

Functional Organizations

Functional organizations are the most common organizations you might see or be involved with. These organizations are organized more by function, such as an information technology (IT) department. A disadvantage of this type of organization is that communication tends to flow from the top down through the organization—from CEO down through the vice presidents (VPs) to the managers, then staff.

A typical functional organization chart might look like the example in Figure 3.4.

Matrix Organizations

A matrix organization takes advantage of staff who might be working on several projects at a time, and therefore would be reporting to both the functional managers and the PMs for their projects.

Within a matrix organization, the power is shared between the two PMs as shown in Figure 3.5.

Project Stakeholder Management

It will be very important to keep key stakeholders involved in the project informed, as a key stakeholder can "make or break" a project. A stakeholder is someone who has a vested interest in the project or can

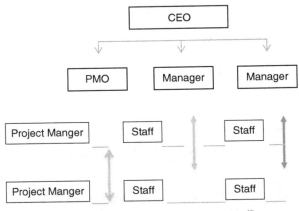

CEO, chief executive officer; PMO, project management office.

FIGURE 3.5 Matrix Organization
From Sipes (2014).

be the greatest critic in the organization. The PM must engage stakeholders, manage expectations, and ensure that the project gets what it needs from stakeholders, and stakeholders get what they need from the project. As the stakeholders are identified, it is important that significant requirements are captured, documented, and incorporated in order to engage stakeholders and manage their expectations. The sooner they are identified, the better the opportunity to gain support and mitigate risks—timely and frequent communication is crucial.

Stakeholders for the project may have different goals. For their departments, they need to meet goals and expectations that will be different from other stakeholders; however, the overall goal of the stakeholders and the project must meet the organization's goals and mission.

There may be three different categories of stakeholders: (a) the project team (internal); (b) stakeholders outside of the project, but within the organization such as the sponsor, functional managers, and organizational groups; and (c) stakeholders outside of the organization, which includes business partners, sellers or suppliers, customers or users, and government regulators.

It will be important to develop a matrix to define which stakeholders own certain parts of the project—include the project team members as this is developed. If important stakeholders are not included in the project, they may not support the project when it is needed or may even interfere with the project—stakeholders' goals may be affected by the project, either positively or negatively, even though they are not actually

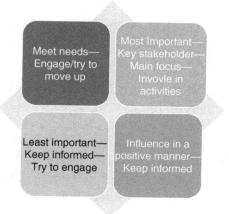

FIGURE 3.6 Stakeholder Analysis
Sipes (2014).

involved in the project. For all of these reasons, it will be crucial to have a documented process for elevating *any* change—that there is a change control board (CCB) and that all changes go through the process.

The team will develop a matrix starting with one side that will reflect those who support the project. There are many examples of matrices available on the web, but a simple example is shown in Figure 3.6.

TEAM SELECTION AND FORMATION

The team members selected for the project will depend on the type of organization and the need for specific applications such as clinical documentation and medication order entry. Team members for these applications include nurses, physicians, and pharmacists. As the teams are formed, necessary skills of potential team members are evaluated. If nurses are needed but the nurses lack analytical skills, they may be sent to the vendor for training. If this type of training—as an analyst—is required, this will need to be added into the project budget.

Organizing teams can be a challenge. Much depends on whether potential members have worked together in the past and, if so, how successful the collaboration was. It would be a big advantage for the advanced practice nurse (APN) if a group of nurses worked together on the same unit and now will work together on a clinical implementation.

As other members are added to the team, there may be more movement through the stages of team formation, which was first described by psychologist Tuckman (1965). The four well-known stages of team development he described are forming, storming, norming, and performing.

- *Forming*—In this first stage, team members are getting to know each other; there is little friction and the team is polite and will offer few opinions. At this stage they do not fully understand what work is required or how each will work together. At this point the PM must be directive and make sure the team has clear objectives. It is also a good time to evaluate individual skills and personalities.
- *Storming*—In the second stage, there may be conflict among team members; there may be challenges to the PM decisions; members may jockey for positions. At this stage, the PM may need to clarify roles if they have not been clear in the past; at this stage authority may be challenged. The APN PMs must remember that they are ultimately responsible for the project.
- *Norming*—In the third stage, the team starts to work better together and resolve their differences; they better understand and respect their different roles as well as those of the PM. As the team moves along and as new tasks come up, there may be periods when they move back to storming as they again clarify their roles. It will be important to facilitate further collaboration among the team members.
- *Performing*—In the fourth stage, the team, without friction, moves toward accomplishing the project goals and objectives. At this point, the APN may more easily delegate much of the work, but must always remember the ultimate responsibility for the entire project lies with the PM (Tuckman, 1965).

An important criterion when leading teams is to establish ground rules at the very start of a project; this will improve team collaboration. Schwarz (2002), an organizational psychologist, suggests that there are eight key rules that effective teams should follow in order to improve team collaboration. The eight ground rules are:

1. State views and ask genuine questions
2. Share all relevant information
3. Use specific examples and agree on what important words mean

4. Explain reasoning and intent
5. Focus on interests, not positions
6. Test assumptions and inferences
7. Jointly design next steps
8. Discuss undiscussable issues (Schwartz, 2002)

The APN as PM should then provide examples and how to use each of these rules. For example, be explicit—say "Put your cell phones on vibrate," "Step out of the room if you must take a call," "Start on time, end on time," "There is no wrong answer," "Treat each other with respect." These are a few of the universal ground rules seen today.

Another researcher, Pentland (2012), looked at data related to team performance and found "with remarkable consistency, the data showed that the most important predictor of a team's success was its communication patterns. Those patterns were as significant as all other factors—intelligence, personality, talent—combined." He identified three communication factors that consistently affect performance: exploration, energy, and engagement. When team members evaluated their own communication styles they found they could dramatically improve their performance.

The APN as PM will invariably find herself or himself in situations of conflict in spite of establishing ground rules. Managing team conflicts is a skill set the APN will need to develop if she or he is not already experienced in resolving conflict. Most of the conflicts will be resolved easily and professionally; it is important to remember that not all conflict is bad. Understanding how to manage conflict will go a long way to dealing with it and must be done to keep the project moving forward.

First, it will be important to determine what caused the conflict, such as prioritizing a task, who should own the task, or trouble with timelines. Once the PM better understands the issues the next step is to get the parties who are having the conflict together. There are several approaches that may lead to conflict resolution: collaboration, compromise, smoothing, withdrawing, as well as others. Each approach has pros and cons, but the key thing to remember is that the project must keep moving on ("Conflict Resolution," 2013). Another process for managing teams is called resource leveling, which is discussed in Chapter 4 on planning.

PM ROLES AND RESPONSIBILITIES

As a PM, the APN will need the skills required to assume the role of PM. Although the APN may not assume a formal PM role, he or she would still apply the project management principles in his or her advanced role as a nurse manager, administrator, quality assurance manager, nursing informaticist, or student in master's and doctoral levels as he or she moves to achieve higher levels of education.

In addition to the skill sets that a PM must have, as discussed earlier, a partial list of classic functions and skills that a PM will be required to have include the ability to:

- Manage teams responsible for delivering the project "outputs" to meet the triple constraints—on time, on budget, in scope
- Plan, organize, monitor, and control the project as a manager
- Handle key responsibilities for developing the project plan and tracking and managing the project, including managing and directing the resources to meet the project objectives; these key responsibilities continue throughout the entire project life cycle
- Continually monitor communications to ensure clear communication with the project team and stakeholders
- Organize the project into small workable steps and monitor closely to ensure all steps are completed to meet project goals
- Design and prepare all project documents, especially scope and charter; obtain all necessary approvals and sign-offs for project deliverables
- Manage stakeholder relationships, including all end user communication and expectations for project tasks
- Work in collaboration with leadership to manage change expectations and behaviors

The project management functions that the APN will be expected to assume are discussed in the next chapters—planning, implementation, monitor and control, and finally closing the project, conducting the final evaluation and lessons learned. Examples of the tools that the APN will need to develop as well as the activities and examples of how to utilize them are included.

SUMMARY

This chapter provides the definitions of the terms that PMs will encounter as they begin to design the project. It provides examples, tables, and figures representative of what is commonly seen in the industry and parallels the expectations of a health care organization, such as the current and future state workflow diagrams, which are created first to determine where gaps in efficiency can be found. It provides examples of a scope document and a charter, which are critical documents that set the boundaries for the project. The SOW description is included because some organizations may require it in addition to the scope and charter documents. Also included is an example of a project timeline that many organizations post for all teams to see. An overview of the organizational structures is provided, as teams and PMs need to understand the hierarchy and management philosophy of the organization.

Finally, team selection and formation criteria are provided, along with typical team behaviors that the APN PM needs to understand in order to have a well-functioning team. The four phases of team behaviors are forming, storming, norming, and performing. There are also suggestions for managing team conflicts and the methods to use to resolve them. Examples of PM roles and responsibilities that may be encountered in a variety of health care settings are also provided. Although PM roles may vary by setting, the project management concepts and principles will always apply. Many explanations and tools provided in this chapter support and help the APN, who is beginning to assume the PM role.

REFERENCES

Banner, C. (2014). *Difference between project charter and project scope.* Retrieved from www.ehow.com

Benjamin, T (n.d.) *What is the difference between a strategic manager & a functional manager?* Retrieved from http://smallbusiness.chron.com/difference-between-strategic-manager-functional-manager-35884.html

Bovend, E., Botell R., & Wade D. (2009). Writing SMART rehabilitation goals and achieving goal attainment scaling: A practical guide. *Clinical Rehabilatation*, 23(4) 352–361. doi:10.1177/0269215508101741

Brief 3: Goals and objectives checklist. (2009). Available at www.cdc.gov/ HealthyYouth/evaluation/resources.htm

Conflict resolution in project management. (2013). Retrieved from http:// programsuccess.wordpress.com

Issel, M. (2004). *Health program planning and evaluation: A practical, systematic approach for community health* (p. 11). Boston, MA: Jones & Bartlett Learning.

Pentland, A. (2012). The new science of building great teams. *Harvard Business Review* (pp. 60–70).

Schwarz, R. (2002). *The skilled facilitator: A comprehensive resource for consultants, facilitators, managers, trainers, and coaches* (4th ed., p. 2). San Francisco, CA: Jossey-Bass.

Sipes, C. (2014). *Developing measureable objectives: Using the five Ws (Document in NR 640, 642 and 643).* Chamberlain College of Nursing, Downers Grove, IL.

Tuckman, B. W. (1965, June). Developmental sequence in small groups. *Psychological Bulletin, 63*(6) 384–399.

CHAPTER 4

Planning:
Project Management—Phase 2

LEARNING OBJECTIVES

Upon completion of this chapter, the reader will be able to:

1. Define the planning phase
2. Discuss three tasks to be accomplished during the planning phase
3. Discuss the value of a work breakdown structure
4. Discuss why a responsibility/accountability matrix is needed
5. Discuss the content documented in the risk plan
6. Define what constraints are. Why do they need to be monitored?
7. Discuss why it is important to define and monitor critical success factors
8. Discuss the value of a network diagram
9. Explain the final step in the planning phase and why it is important

OUTLINE

- Key Terms
- Introduction
- Statement of Work (SOW)
- The Project Plan
- Work Breakdown Structure
- Tracking Schedules
- Building the Budget and Managing the Resources

- Project Responsibility and Accountability
- Risk Assessment and Management Plan
- Communication
- Change Management
- Deliverables and Critical Success Factors (CSF)
- Status Meetings
- Kick-Off Meeting

KEY TERMS

Actual cost of work performed (ACWP)

Budgeted cost of work performed (BCWS)

Budgeted cost of work scheduled (BCWP)

Change management

Constraints

Cost variance (CV)

Critical path (CP)

Critical success factors (CSF)

Deliverables

Earned value (EV)

Fast Track

Gantt chart

Kick-off meeting

Network diagram

Responsible, accountable, consulted, informed (RACI)

Risk

Schedule variance (SV)

Statement of work (SOW)

Status meetings

Work breakdown structure (WBS)

INTRODUCTION

Planning Processes, Tools, and Skills Needed for the Project

After the design/initiation phase of project management comes the second, or planning, phase of a project. If the project has been approved and the key stakeholders have signed off on it, it means there is support for the planning and implementation of the project. This phase is one of the most important phases of the project. If tasks or activities are not identified and planned during this phase, it can cause delays in the overall project. If the advanced practice nurse project manager (APN PM) does not develop the plan with great detail it may be one of the reasons for project delay, even failure, especially if a key task was forgotten. Many times senior leadership are anxious to move quickly to implement a project and cut the planning phase short, which may create a potential gap in the planning process. The detailed, very specific project plan is key to setting the expectations for the five Ws and an H (Sipes, 2014): who, what, where, why, when, and how of a project. All of these specific details were outlined in the project objectives during the design phase and now will be revised.

Eight Steps in Project Planning

The planning steps of project management are like a road map that gives the detail necessary for the PM to support the project team so that it thrives, while the PM helps the team navigate the project highway and close a successful project. Many of the project tasks or items build upon one another. They are not set in stone. They can be changed, using the process and tools you will develop in this phase when you create the change management plan. Many of the tools and different variations of tools can be found on the web. Most organizations define their own model of how they want a project completed and have tools unique to their organization as well.

The project's scope and charter are developed and approved during the inital phase, that is, design/initiation. The planning phase then builds on the processes established in the design phase and now will develop the work breakdown structure (WBS) and schedules using the eight steps in project planning, which are:

1. Build a project scope based upon the project charter.
2. Breakdown the scope into tasks/work packages.
3. Assign tasks/work packages to their owners.
4. Task/Work package owners build activity lists.
5. Activity owners estimate or calculate activity durations.
6. As a team, activity owners sequence activities.
7. Identify and document dependencies.
8. Build a schedule based on steps 1–7.

It will be important to know which tools should be developed first, then others may follow the same format making each subsequent tool easier and more efficient to build. Project teams often struggle with the level of detail in the tools and documents such as the charter saying, they cannot build it yet, because they do not know enough about the project. It is important to remember that documents and tools developed are not set in stone. Changes can be made as new information becomes available, as long as the change management process and tracking tools are used. You are learning that project planning is critical to a project's success and extremely important for the project team. To be effective and efficient a team must have a plan. Without a plan to provide structure and direction, a project can become lost, inadvertently consuming resources and jeopardizing the triple constraints. The amount of detail in the plan and the number of components in the plan vary depending on several factors: project duration, project complexity, and organizational adherence to a formal project management methodology. To reinforce what was learned in Chapter 3—Design/Initiation—the emphasis is on SMART objectives or the five Ws for measureable objectives, which should be very detailed in order to provide direction for the project.

Support Documents

The support documents and tools that should be developed during the planning phase include but are not limited to:

- A WBS
- Project plan with Gantt chart
- Network diagram
- Project schedules
- Communication plan
- Risk-management plan
- Resource management plan

The project charter was created and approved in Chapter 3. The other project tools are developed by the project team and approved by all of the key project stakeholders unless the organization has its own tools and documents that will be required. The approval process is very important because it officially authorizes the use of resources for the project.

Effective project teams take this approval one step further by performing a baseline assessment. The baseline is a snapshot, a static picture of the project. It is essentially the APN PM's estimates of:

- Tasks
- Resources
- Start dates
- End dates
- Completion date
- Budgets or costs

This baseline is essential for tracking because it serves as a reference or benchmark with which you can monitor your project's performance. You can compare your planning against the actual results of your project. Once you have a baseline, future changes must undergo the change management process discussed later in this chapter, and all comparisons (variances) are based on the baseline values. Recall the triple constraints. The budget, requirements, and schedule are the project tools and processes that are most frequently base lined.

There are times when leadership, especially on a new project, does not value the time and amount of planning that is required at this point in the project's continuum, but the level of detail in the project documents and tools is critical and will ultimately save time later because some important step was not overlooked. It is important to remember that planning is strongly associated with project success. Again, the primary function of a project plan is to give the PM a map of the route from project start to finish. The APN PM will use the key documents noted here as well as those from Chapter 3, to create this map. The map should contain sufficient information so that at any time the PM knows what remains to be done, when and with what resources the tasks will be completed, and what objectives the project is supposed to meet.

Key Components of a Project Plan

There are many techniques for developing a project plan, and they are fundamentally similar. You need to develop a systematic analysis to identify and list what must be done in order to achieve the project's objectives, to test and validate the plan, and to deliver it to your stakeholders. This process was started when the needs assessment and gap analysis was completed in Chapter 3. The key components of the project plan discussed and demonstrated in this chapter are:

- The project plan or resource management plan (work plan) and Gantt chart
- The WBS
- The project schedules, including network diagram, critical path
- The risk management plan
- The communication plan
- Change management plan
- Status meetings

During the design and planning phases—the first two phases—most of the documents and tools needed during the implementation of the project will be developed. The deliverables and documents needed to start the project include a scope and charter, project plan using a Gantt chart, WBS, network diagram, cost estimates, RACI (responsible, accountable, consulted, informed), risk management tool, communication and change management plans, timeline chart, identification and documentation constraints, project deliverables defined, and status meeting processes, documents and other tracking tools.

As the project moves forward toward implementation, a final step for phase 2 is the kick-off meeting, which essentially launches the implementation and energizes the team as they start the next and longest phase of the project—implementation phase. This phase will also add more clarity for the team as they begin to see more structure added to the project as well as clarity to their roles.

STATEMENT OF WORK (SOW)

An important note here is that if you are working in a larger organization or project management office (PMO), you may be expected to create a SOW. A SOW is a document that will outline the project or service, the timeline for expected completion, deliverables, and assumptions. It also defines how the project should proceed and vendor, if included, expectations and timeline for completion. More frequently today this information is included in the detail of the scope and charter documents as well as the WBS and project plan. This is another reason it is very important to add detail and be very specific when developing your project documents and preparing weekly and monthly status reports. This is mentioned here only so that you understand some of the terminology that can be checked further if applicable.

THE PROJECT PLAN

Previously, you may have thought that a project plan was a schedule—they are different. A schedule is part of the project plan that would not succeed without one. The schedule in the project plan defines the due dates for different tasks that need to be completed. There are several types of schedules that will be discussed later. Schedules are critically important in that they can graphically display the project plan and allows a quick overview of the project, owners and due dates.

One of the first things you will do as the APN PM is to create a project plan is. It is very important to remember that any task that was started without a plan and due diligence is almost always doomed as a failure from the start. In the previous chapter, you defined the scope, developed SMART objectives or the five Ws and H for measurable objectives, and identified the stakeholders who approved the project. Now you will add some of that content to the project plan.

Deliverables

Preliminary lists of project deliverables are to be created in the scope and charter as described in Chapter 3. Now that more information is available, you will be able to more clearly define the project deliverables. Deliverables are the items needed to meet the goals and objectives of the project. As you did when creating your measurable objectives, add to your project charter the dates when these items are due and define how they will be delivered. Remember, the due dates can be adjusted as the schedules are put together. Start by creating the task list of items needed to meet the project deliverables. As the task list is created, add the estimated hours it will take to complete the task and the owner responsible. The work packages or tasks are unique because they are each a deliverable; again, remember that you may need to revise the list as more information becomes available.

Project Scheduling

One definition of a schedule is that it is the conversion of a project action plan into an operating timetable where it will become the basis for monitoring and controlling project activity. This chapter provides a closer look at the different types of project schedules that will be needed on the project. Examples are provided on how to break what are called tasks/work packages from the WBS down into smaller parts or tasks, then, organize the tasks into a schedule.

First, it is important to understand the scheduling terminology and then learn how to take a simple plan and schedule tasks from the WBS manually using network diagrams. Many times organizations provide software, such as Microsoft Project, so that scheduling can be completed by the PM or designate. The different types of schedules are discussed here but first an understanding of the WBS that will be used to develop the schedules is needed.

WORK BREAKDOWN STRUCTURE

The WBS is developed to show in detail the work and specific tasks that need to be completed before the project can be considered ready to implement. However, it is not the project plan or schedule. This is one of the first project documents you will need to develop and it is key to going forward with your project plan. There are a number of different guidelines for the size of the tasks. The most universal one is to break down the scope into pieces of work that will be assigned an owner. You must first fully understand exactly which tasks and activities need to be completed. It will help you see the detail of the project in smaller, workable, more manageable components (see Figure 4.1). The WBS is typically completed before the Gantt charts are developed, as it is the first document to essentially divide the project into smaller tasks. If a task seems too large to manage, it is an indication that they need to be broken down into smaller activities or if too small can lead to micromanagement of the activity. It will give you and your stakeholders a quick view of the project requirements and a view of what tasks will need to be accomplished in each of the five phases of the project.

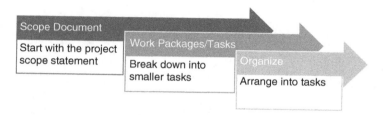

FIGURE 4.1 Steps to Developing a Work Breakdown Structure (WBS)

The WBS graphical view shown in Figure 4.2 represents how the work packages or tasks can be broken down into tasks and sub-tasks. The columns show the WBS code (1; 1.1) and activities. WBS codes are numbered and indented so that the level of each activity or task is clearly identified. This example represents Project XYZ, which has been funded by a health care organization. The figure shows five phases of the project. The five phases of all project management projects are discussed in Chapters 3 to 7. The tasks for each phase of the project include:

- Phase 1—Design/Initiate—Four of the tasks to be completed in this phase include developing the charter and scope, conducting the needs assessment, and developing the objectives (Chapter 3).
- Phase 2—Planning—A partial list of the tasks to be completed during this phase include developing the project plan, WBS, risk plans, assigning the project team, and kick-off (Chapter 4).
- Phase 3—Implement/Execution—The tasks to be completed in this phase include implementing the project, creating the change management and risks plans, and holding the status meetings (Chapter 5).
- Phase 4—Monitor and Control—The tasks to be completed in this phase include change control, monitoring risk, controlling the schedule, and monitoring costs. It is important to remember that the monitor and control functions overlap the implementation as that is where the processes are originally employed—to monitor and control the implementation (Chapter 6).
- Phase 5—Close and Evaluate—The tasks to be completed in this phase include obtaining project verification, conducting a lessons learned analysis, obtaining final acceptance, and transitioning the project to leadership. This example in Figure 4.2 is only representation of a few of the tasks needed to complete a project—the one the APN PM will develop will include much more detail (Chapter 7).

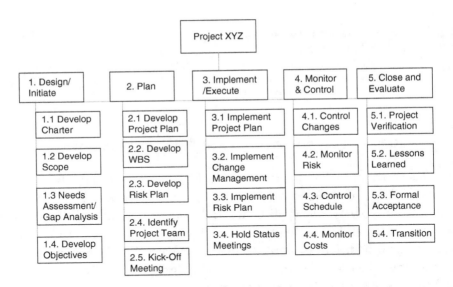

FIGURE 4.2 Work Breakdown Structure (WBS)—Graphical Version
From Sipes (2014).

Work Packages/Tasks

After the scope statement has been approved, the team begins to identify the work packages/tasks that must be completed to deliver the project's scope. A work package is a deliverable or a subset of a project; it can be thought of as a miniature project within the large project or a piece of the WBS. The work packages are unique because they are each a deliverable; they make the work manageable because the APN PM can detail the steps needed to complete each work package. All of the work packages or miniature projects combine to complete the entire project. This allows the teams to work on their work packages or deliverables concurrently if necessary.

One of the first steps to identify work packages or tasks is to hold a brainstorming session with the project team. Then the tasks are collected and documented in the WBS. Using the scope statement, the project is decomposed/broken down into smaller work packages. The end goal is to identify each task at the most granular and detailed level where the work can be recognized by the stakeholders. The smaller and more detailed task help to facilitate control of the project and improve communication about the project. Finally, after the WBS tasks have been defined with great detail, the next step will be to develop the RACI that will define duties and responsibilities.

TRACKING SCHEDULES

There are different types of schedules including the network diagram and critical path. Network diagrams are a "schematic display of the logical relationships" and sequence of activities (Microsoft, 2014) that provides a quick view of the tasks needed to be completed with a particular project. The network diagram enables the APN PM to determine the schedule times for related project activities, the critical path of the project, and the float or slack time (the amount of time that an activity may be delayed without delaying the project).

Why Build a Network Diagram?

One of the most important aspects of project management is building a project schedule. An important tool called a network diagram is a great way to track the project tasks and provides a quick visual of what needs to be done. There are two good reasons to learn how to develop this tool:

1. Today most organizations use network diagrams in some form or another
2. It is an industry standard.

There are several ways to build a network diagram; one way will be to use the activity in box (AIB) method (network diagraming) also known as activity on node (AON)—they are the same. With this concept, you will be able to determine (1) a project's scheduled completion time, (2) the slack or float time of project activities, and (3) the critical path of your project (for examples, see "Definition of Activity in a Box," 2014)

Microsoft Project can make it easy to build a network diagram. It is like adding—you should first do it manually for simple diagrams and critical paths but when it is more complex use a calculator. Every PM should know how to build a network diagram manually so that he or she really understands the concepts before working in Microsoft Project. The APN PMs who understand it are much more effective and know how to use the tools more effectively. Those who do not know how to build a schedule manually often make mistakes and negatively impact a project's triple constraints. Practice is required for proficiency.

To Build a Network Diagram

After the tasks in the WBS are created, they are assigned to the people, or teams of people, who are responsible for delivering the tasks, in a step-by-step process. One way to start building a network diagram is to brainstorm with the project team that will record all of the tasks on sticky notes (without regard to sequencing). Then start listing the tasks in the order they should occur, determine which activities can occur at the same time, and which activities need dependencies—which means one task must be completed before the next can be started (e.g. medical orders must be defined and updated before they can be built), if a task is considered discretionary—that is, it is determined as a best practice or convenience and may have to wait. However, the subsequent task can begin if the secondary dependency is not completed.

After all of the tasks have been defined, put the notes on a wall after writing in the earlier information then start to build a network using the notes. If building a more complex network diagram, a second row can be laid out horizontally along with the original row. It will be very important to start out simply before moving to a more complex diagram.

Next, the activities are assigned to the people who will be doing the work. The team will build duration estimates for the activities. It is important to work as a team since many tasks are dependent on other activities in the team. The most accurate estimates are built using actual data from previous, similar projects if available. Then the activities can be loaded into an automated scheduling tool such as Microsoft Project. At that point, you will be able to determine the project's scheduled completion time, the slack or float of project activities, and the critical path of your project. As mentioned, it is also important to be able to build such a network manually; you will better understand the concepts after you have done this. See the network diagram and critical path example in Figure 4.3.

More Terminology

As you develop the network diagram, you will also need to lay out the critical path. The critical path analysis or method (CPM) represents the tasks or activities that have float or slack of 0 days, which means they cannot be delayed without delaying the entire project—they are the critical tasks. Advantages to using the CPM are that it defines which tasks must be completed and which can be done in parallel. It also

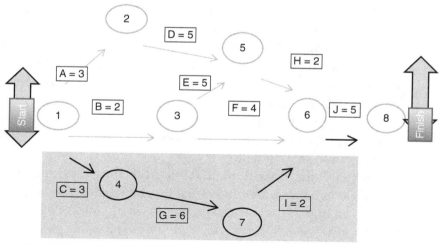

Path 1: A-D-H-J = 3 days + 5 + 2 + 5 = 15 days (1 > 2 > 5 > 6 > 8)

Path 2: B-E-F-J = 2 days + 4 + 5 = 11 days (1 > 3 > 6 > 8)

Path 3: B-E-H-J = 2 days + 5 + 2 + 5 = 14 days (1 > 3 > 5 > 6 > 8)

Path 4: C-G-I-J = 3 days + 6 + 2 + 5 = 16 days (1 > 4 > 7 > 6 > 8)—Critical Path

FIGURE 4.3 Network Diagram With Critical Path

helps to visualize the shortest and longest time to complete the project and where the resources are needed as the activities are defined along a line showing how they will sequence and follow. Using the CPM can help make a project more successful as the detailed activities are more clearly defined and tracked (see Figure 4.3).

Other important terms to understand include:

- AIB is the same as a network diagram—it is a graphical representation of the activities that need to be competed
- AON—Activity on node, the nodes are the boxes such as "start"
- Early start (ES) = The earliest time the activity could possibly start
- Early finish (EF) = The earliest time the activity or project could possibly finish
- Late start (LS) = The latest time the activity can start and not jeopardize the scheduled completion of the project
- Late finish (LF) = The latest time the activity can finish without causing the project to be late

- Slack or float for each activity. Slack/float is determined by LF – EF or the time between the ES – LS. The slack/float tells you the number of days, weeks, or months that an activity can begin late or the number of extra days, weeks, or months that an activity can take without delaying a succeeding activity or impacting the completion time of the project. Float is the "extra" cushion time built into a project that will not actually cause a delay in the project, as you anticipate that projects are always delayed to some extent.
- Crashing the critical path (CP)—This means adding more resources to activities to get them completed earlier. Caution: CP will impact budget and quality—two of your constraints.
- Fast tracking—Perform more activities in parallel
- Resource leveling—Adding resources with related activities to the same process; this may cause bottlenecks due to resources being unavailable for other activities.
- PERT (Program Evaluation and Review Technique) PERT is a variation on the CPM. It is a more rigorous approach and uses a statistical formula to calculate time estimates. There are tutorials available to develop this skill if the organization requires this scheduling method.
- Milestone—In the network diagram a milestone is represented by the node or box. These are also the deliverables discussed earlier in this chapter and are also listed in the project scope and charter documents discussed in Chapter 3.

The CP is the longest path through the diagram in Figure 4.3, which is 16 days—the path and arrows in gray. The critical path is the longest time tasks on the path can be completed and already has some slack/float built in. Figure 4.3 is only representative of certain tasks and not all on the project; for example, the build of a clinical documentation application. It also shows which tasks must be completed before the next tasks. For example task 1—if you were doing a workflow analysis—has to be completed before the medical orders—tasks 4, 7, 6, 8—can be built and so on.

There are many tutorials available to practice and polish the skills discussed in this chapter that are needed to be successful as a PM. You will find these listed the References section of this chapter.

Critical success factors (CSF) for the CPM involve tracking the critical tasks and resources; this will determine which tasks affect the project's finish date and whether the project will finish on time.

BUILDING THE BUDGET AND MANAGING THE RESOURCES

Developing the budget is one of the most important tasks the APN PM will accomplish. Budget management involves the creation and monitoring of a project budget, and identifying, reporting and escalating variances if they are out of line—moving beyond 5% over the original budget. Tracking coasts and resource consumption closely throughout the project is critical and one of the most important tasks a PM will accomplish. The chief finance officer (CFO) will be the primary contact for the more complex budget tasks as PMs are not expected to be experts in budget development and management but must be knowable of basic concepts that are described here. Basic terminology and sample budgets can be found here.

Determining Cost Estimates—Cost Analysis Tools

Other tools the APN PM can use to manage costs and budgets are exception reporting and calculating earned value (EV). You use cost variance (CV), schedule variance (SV), and indexes to help focus on the activities that are in danger of not being met or of going over budget. The monitoring and control of costs is one of the key tasks to follow as the project is implemented. The calculation of these values can also be done using a software package such as Microsoft Project.

EV Analysis

In order to calculate CV and SV, you will need three very important numbers for each activity. A few important terms to know before beginning to calculate the EV are BCWS, BCWP, and ACWP. The formula is BCWP − ACWP = BCWS or your actual budget. This should not be a negative number, which would indicate being over budget.

- BCWS = budgeted cost of work scheduled
- BCWP = budgeted cost of work performed (also called EV)— will change throughout the project
- ACWP = actual cost of work performed—will change throughout the project

An example of what this might look like:

Table 4.1 shows what a partially completed Gantt chart might look like (originally formatted in Excel). The left side of diagram is a tabular structure, with 7 rows, and 8 columns. The column headings are (1) Number of Task, (2) Task Name, (3) Duration, and (4) Resource Names to be added. To the right of the Resource /Owner is a graphing area where the duration of the tasks are illustrated with solid lines. The headings in the graphing section are from left to right, are in weeks indicating the estimated length of the task by week—this can also be designed by months.

1. Row **1.** = Task Name – **Design Project**. The task bar's left edge starts in Oct 27 and extends to 15 days – Bold indicates major tasks; tasks listed under the major task are sub-tasks.
2. Row 1.1 = Task Name – General Contractor. The task bar's left edge starts on Oct 27 and extends 4 days.
3. Row 1.2 = Task Name – Hire Subcontractor. The task bar's left edge starts on Oct 27 and extends 4 days.
4. Row 1.3 = Task Name – Develop Foundation Plans. The task bar's left edge starts on Oct 27 and extends 6 days.
5. Row **2** = Task Name – **Frame and Pour Foundation.** The task bar's left edge starts on Oct 27 and extends for 25 days.

TABLE 4.1
Sample: Basic Budget Preparation

Task Number	Task Name	Task Duration	Resource/ Owner	27-Oct	3-Nov	10-Nov	17-Nov
1	**Design Project**	**15 days**					
1.1	Hire general contractor	4 days					
1.2	Hire subcontractor	4 days					
1.3	Develop foundation plans	6 days					
2	**Frame and Pour Foundation**	**25 days**					
2.1	Finish basement prep	7 days					
2.2	Add drainage around foundation	2 days					

From Sipes (2014).

6. Row 2.1 = Task Name – Finish Basement Prep. The task bar's left edge starts on Oct 27 and extends for 7 days.
7. Row 2.2 = Task Name – Add Drainage Around Foundation. The task bar's left edge starts on Oct 27 and extends 2 days.

Sample Budget: Assume Budget is:

Design Project – $5,000
General Contractor – $25,000
Hire Subcontractor – $15,000
Develop Foundation Plans – **$500**
Frame and Pour Foundation – $18,000
Finish Basement Prep – $8,000
Add Drainage Around Foundation – $400

In Week 1, you finalized 40% of the design for the project. In Week 2, you hired the general contractor and revised/updated the project plan and grade the building site. Both of those activities are scheduled to take 4 days. For these exercises, you assume costs are even across time.

BCWS for Week 1 = 40% × $5,000 = $2,000
BCWS for Week 2 = 60% ($5,000) + 25% ($25,000) + 30% (15,000) + 70% (500) = $14,100 to get project started.
Budget costs accumulate over the life of a project. Therefore, Week 1 and 2's costs are added into Week 3's costs and so on.

TABLE 4.2
Summary of Initial Work Completed

Activity	WK 1	WK 2	WK 3	WK 4
Design project	40%	60%	100%	
Hire general contractor		25%		
Hire subcontractor		30%		25%
Develop foundation plans		20%		
Pour foundation				
Pour basement				
Arrange drainage around foundation				

BCWS for Week 3 = (100 − 60 = 40% due left on designing project)
40% × 5,000 = $2,000 (Total to date: $18,100)
BCWS for Week 4 = 25% × (15,000) = $3,750 as the subcontract or
has asked for an advance on salary

In the example Table 4.2—look at the actual costs by week. In this case ACWP are exactly what was budgeted.

ACWP for Week 1 = 40% × $5,000 = $2,000
ACWP for Week 2 = 60% ($5,000) + 25% ($25,000) + 30% ($15,000) + 70% ($500) = $14,100 to get project started.
Budget costs accumulate over the life of a project. Therefore, Week 1 and 2's costs are added into budget costs accumulated over the life of a project, but the percentages in the chart build in that accumulation for you.
ACWP for Week 3 = (100 − 60 = 40% due left on designing project) 40% × 5,000 = $2,000. (Total to date: $18,100)
ACWP for Week 4 = 25% × ($15,000) = $3,750

Again, ACWP cannot be calculated until after work begins. In this case you have not calculated how the budget and actual costs are aligned until Week 4 as you are preparing a month-end report for the senior vice president and one of the key stakeholders. This calculation is not difficult; just add up the bills and salaries.

A third calculation is the BCWP. In this case the BCWS + the ACWP + the BCWP are all in agreement. An example of when this might not be the case is when the work scheduled falls behind and more temporary resources are hired to get the project back on track. Then both the *actual* and *budgeted* cost of the work performed would be over budget. BCWP − ACWP should not be a negative number—if so the project is over budget.

Another consideration most companies use a "loaded rate" to account for pension plans, insurance, and so forth. A loaded rate or a loaded labor rate links variable overhead, fixed overhead costs, and net profit with a unit of labor such as wage or salary. For example, a loaded rate might have an additional 15% to 20% added to cover salary or wages + benefits + overhead costs + profit margin and also include equipment costs and supplies and overhead or operating costs. Some examples might include rent, electricity, gas, water, and sewage. Once you have completed the BCWS, BCWP and ACWP, the rest of EV analysis is simply plugging in the numbers.

More Terminology

The EV is the budgeted cost of work that has been completed to date of review (current date). EV can also include finished components of a work product. EV is established by the planned costs and the rate that the team is completing the work to date. Another term is CV, which is the difference between the work that has been completed (in dollars) and how much was spent to accomplish this work. For example: CV = EV – actual cost; another example: CV = BCWP (work performed) – ACWP. A negative result means you are over budget. If you budgeted 20 hours and the actual work was 36 hours = 16 hours were not budgeted.

A SV is the difference between what was planned and what has actually been done to date. For example: SV—BCWP—BCWS; you have planned that the "Finish basement prep" was going to take 7 days, but it snowed so that the basement prep took 14 days. The budgeted plan of the work performed was only partially completed in the time budgeted—7 days versus 14 days = –7 days over schedule—you are behind schedule.

More Considerations

Being on time and budget are emphasized as doing a great job managing the project. However, if a project is reporting cost and SVs that are always too favorable, it could be an indication that work is not being performed with high quality, or the efforts have been overestimated. If the project is reporting CVs or SVs that are too negative, it means that something is amiss, or the efforts have been underestimated. The sooner the variances are reviewed, the quicker corrective action can be taken. Some projects use variance levels as triggers to alert management to potential oversight. Too much variance in either direction should be

TABLE 4.3
Example: Owners/Team Members and Hours Budgeted to Work on Project

Resource Name			Work to Date		
Joe Smith			Budgeted 1,032 hrs.		
Task Name	Units	Work	Delay	Start	Finish
Analyze workflow	100%	24 hrs.	0 hrs.	Mon 10/8/01	Wed 10/10/01
Team meetings; every 2 weeks	100%	4 hrs.	0 hrs.	Thu 10/11/01	Thu 10/17//01
Start Clinc Doc build	100%	16 hrs.	0 hrs.	Thu 10/11/01	Fri 10/13/01

closely reviewed. The APN PM must determine how much oversight is necessary based on the needs of each project.

Estimating Costs

In addition to the methods in Table 4.3, there are several other types of budgeting. Many organizations use a combination of strategies, depending on where they are in the life cycle of a project. It is important for the APN PM to have basic understanding of some of the terminology.

Fixed costs ("fixed costs and variable costs," n.d.) are costs that remain constant regardless of the duration of a project or scale of business activity. For example, a purchase of a crane or computer system is the same cost regardless of the duration of the project.

Variable costs ("fixed costs and variable costs," n.d.) are costs that vary with time or resource changes. For example, labor costs are dependent on the number of hours worked. An example of how you might put the owners/team members and hours each is expected to work on a project is provided in Table 4.3.

To Crash a Budget

Crashing a budget refers to a management method for shortening the duration of a project by decreasing the time it takes to complete one or more of the project's activities. In some types of projects, there are standard crash costs formulas that PMs can use to determine how a project's budget would be affected by crashing an activity or activities. Typically the activities that are reduced are critical activities.

For example, in a clinical documentation project the analyst can use a standard generic application used on other projects or do a custom build. In this example, the normal time would be 3 days, with a total normal cost of $300 ($100 per day) to implement the build of the custom application. The crash time would be 1 day to implement the generic application; the total crash cost would be $600. To determine the crash cost difference: 3 days @ $100 day = $300 versus 1 day @ $600 = saving 2 days on the project timeline but $300 over budget. What is the value of doing this? All constraints need to be analyzed for the best approach. This would be an important issue to discuss with leadership including the sponsor. This is a very simple example; most are much more complex but it provides an example of the concept.

PROJECT RESPONSIBILITY AND ACCOUNTABILITY

Assigning Responsibility

The responsibility assignment matrix (RAM) is an excellent way to clearly assign all of the WBS tasks to a person or another team.The purpose of a RAM document—sometimes referred to as the RACI—is to identify who "owns" a specific task or activity as well as the person who is accountable and will sign off on the task when it is completed. To complete the RAM/RACI, first identify all of the project tasks and activities that need to be completed before the project can be implemented. This also includes deliverables and milestones previously identified. Although responsibility can be shared, each activity or task should have only one person responsible as owner, otherwise it may cause issues of ownership. RACI stands for:

- R = Responsible—the person who does the work
- A = Accountable—the person who must ensure that the work is completed (often the PM)
- C = Consulted—this person often has information required to complete the work package
- I = Informed—this is often the largest group and typically includes all of the key stakeholders

TABLE 4.4
Responsibility Matrix—RACI

Project Task/ Activities	Project Manager / Owner of Task = R = Joe	Approve Accountable/ Sign-Off = A = Bob	Consulted re: Work Product = C = Jim	Informed/ Notified of Results = I = Sue
Develop scope	R	A	C	I
Develop charter	R	A	C	I
Team selection	A	R	C	I
Communication plan	R	I	I	I
Risk plan	R	I	I	I
Change control plan	R	I	I	I
Weekly status meetings	R	I	I	I

R = responsible; A = accountable; C = consulted; I = informed.

As an example and using a few of the tasks from the WBS, Table 4.4 is an excerpt from the project development process. It is important to note that the responsibilities can vary depending on the project. For example, the PM generally takes responsibility for the scope and charter documents, whereas, in other areas the team selection will require responsibility from Bob—a key stakeholder.

RISK ASSESSMENT AND MANAGEMENT PLAN

Risk is anything that can negatively or positively impact the project. One positive impact that we see is a vendor who supplies product to us before it was expected. This positively impacted the project and helped the project to be completed ahead of schedule. Other risks can negatively impact the project. Not all risks that are identified will occur, but because they can, we must manage them. A risk management plan states how risks will be identified, assessed, and managed during the project life cycle. The APN PM must be sure that at least the five steps here are analyzed—there may be more needed but this is the basic process to follow. Then develop the risk management plan documenting responses to the five steps here.

- Identify Risk—Internal and external including vendors; what are the skill levels of all
- Asses Risk—Prioritize low, medium, high

- Manage Risk—Determine—Remove, shift, and decrease impact; re-assess
- Monitor and Control Each Risk—For higher risk, implement more frequent monitoring
- Establish an Ongoing Management Plan for Risk Assessment— that requires constant review; update and remove those risks not impacting project

The process of risk management identifies all positive and negative risks to a project. It is through the risk management plan that the APN as PM will be able to address and document all risks that could affect the project. Frequent risk reviews keep a focus on risks as they arise, then are managed.

All projects have some risk, especially when you have more people involved, which can cause confusion about what needs to be done and when it is due. That is why it is very important to document all risks that could potentially impact the project, whether large or small, even though they seem harmless or will not impact any other task. This includes all people, processes, technology, environmental influences, and organizational processes. Conducting and updating a risk assessment must be be ongoing throughout the entire project. Potential risk areas that must be continually monitored are the triple constraints—time, cost/under-budgeted, resources not committed/lacking anticipated skill as well as:

- Any budget cuts
- Role confusion—unclear/undefined responsibilities
- Lack of stakeholder or leadership support
- Poor communication

These and all other risks will need to be tracked closely on the risk plan shown in Table 4.5. You will need to write down what you will do in the event it does occur and what you will do to prevent the occurrence. This should be reviewed with the project team at the weekly team and stakeholder meetings. Risks that are labeled as "high" should be addressed immediately as it may delay the forward progress of the project.

Content for each column in Table 4.6

- Rank each risk: highest probability at the top
- Add source of risk: risk trigger; resolution if triggered
- Rate: high, medium, low
- Impact on project

TABLE 4.5
Sample: Risk Analysis Document and Plan

| | | | Version: | | | | | Date: | | |
No.	Rank	Category	Risk	Description	Triggers	Potential Responses	Probability	Impact	Risk Owner	Status/Was issue escalated? Y/N
1		Med orders application	High	Not built correctly—does not interface	Nurses documenting med orders	Med orders do not show	High	High	Project manager, Willow	PM, Willow, IT, In review—Y
	2		High							
	3		Med							
	4		Low							

TABLE 4.6

Examples of Change Management Log From the CDC

Project Name: <optional>
National Center: <required>
Project Manager Name: <required>
Project Description: <required>

ID	Current Status	Priority	Change Request Description	Assigned to Owner	Expected Resolution Date	Escalation Required (Y/N)?	Action Steps
	Open	Critical	**EXAMPLE:** Request for product functionality increase			Yes	**EXAMPLE:** Analyze impact of requested change and then meet with the change control board (CCB) to present findings for final decision on the requested change
	Work In Progress	High	**EXAMPLE:** The schedule slipped due to unexpected weather-related events			No	**EXAMPLE:** Adjust the schedule to account for the weather-related events
	Closed	Medium					
		Low					

Adapted www2a.cdc.gov (2014).

- Risk owner: who will be responsible if risk occurs
- Current status of risk
- Category: where the risk is in relation to other tasks in the project

Critical success factors related to risk management include:

- Issue is resolved quickly and accurately
- All issues are documented and tracked with action plans
- Document of the issue management exists with owners and due dates
- Communication of key issues is completed and documents the who, what, why, where, and when.

Finally, all risk mitigation plans and the success of the plan as well as next steps will need to be documented. It is important that the risks are quickly identified before they impact project milestones.

COMMUNICATION

Communication is a key aspect throughout a project. All stakeholders must effectively communicate throughout the project's life cycle. A good project plan with poor communication—or a poor project plan with good communication—is ineffective and can lead to project failure. Think of an example of a successful team—football team, other teams, a team at work. Why are these teams successful or unsuccessful? When comparing the two types of teams, think about the people on the teams. It is not the uniform or equipment but the people. Good communication with the people on the teams is the key to a project success. Communication is an extremely important skill and a key tool for a PM. Knowing who your stakeholders are and making sure you communicate with them effectively and efficiently is a skill common to successful PMs.

Organizations have many formats for a communication plan. Reflect on the formats used at your institution Communication can take many forms. Written, oral, listening, and nonverbal cues are typical means of communication. It is important that communication approaches are made up of a two-way approach. Some examples are speaking and listening, writing and reading, and sending and receiving messages. Organizational structures can have different communication forms,

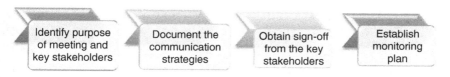

FIGURE 4.4 Steps to Developing a Communication Plan

such as internal, external, vertical, and horizontal. Finally, there are informal and formal communication forms.

Steps that outline how to build a communication plan are listed in Figure 4.4. Communication plans are an excellent resource for any groups of people who communicate. If you use the four steps in Figure 4.4, or develop a different one, the key thing to remember is that you do need a framework communication plan that will always be consistent in format; people will begin to expect it on a weekly or regular basis.

Project communication includes meetings, status reports, presentations at different steering team meetings such as executive steering team (EST) and project steering team (PST) meetings, and documentation in a project notebook. It is important to remember that your communications must be succinct and to the point. If the EST and other stakeholders are frequently sent unnecessary information they will stop reading the updates, which they may view as a waste of time. Something to remember is to focus on getting the right information to the right people at the right time.

It is very important for PMs to be effective communicators. Clear, concise, succinct, and timely communication can add clarity to a complex project. As previously discussed, projects can be matrix, functional, or project structured and, in each case, a PM must be able to effectively communicate across geographic, technical, and business boundaries. From another perspective, a PM with good communication skills can help an ailing project. Conversely, a PM with poor communication skills can erode the focus of the project and jeopardize one or more of the triple constraints.

CHANGE MANAGEMENT

Change management is difficult because most people do not do it right. "According to a 2013 Strategy/Katzenbach Center Survey of global senior executives on culture and change management, the success rate of major change initiatives is only 54 percent" ... which is far too low (as cited in Aguirre & Alpern, 2014, p. 3). As PM, you must embrace change as a good thing, keep everyone in the loop, and get necessary approvals on requested changes to move them to accept changes. The PM and stakeholders champion this effort. There are several ways project change can occur. The project stakeholders may request to change the original approved project scope, or they may want to extend the project schedule, the budget may have been underestimated, the technology was not completely understood, or even a new law or mandate was passed.

Changes to the scope may require a phased approach where portions of the scope are moved to a second or third phase. There are times when the PM must negotiate for more time. The impact of a scheduling change can be far reaching because it affects the budget and many people, including paid contractors and vendors, as well as employees whose commitment to the project has expired. Time extensions are a negative reflection on the PM and should be avoided.

Some of the most difficult changes occur when there has been an assumption or misunderstanding of what was to occur. If this happens, the easiest approach is to go back and carefully list all of the assumptions, including technology, and review if the assumptions are still relevant. If not they all need to be revised as well as the project schedule and budget. For change to be effective, it must be clear and determined through collaboration with all stakeholders and decision makers, and everyone must be committed to the change.

The Katzenback Center identified 10 principles for change that they recommend should be used as guidelines when anticipating change. These include:

1. Lead with the culture—determine where the resistance is, how do people behave, how are decisions made
2. Engage employees at all levels but start at the top to get support
3. Involve every layer
4. Make the rational and emotional case together
5. Act your way into new thinking—evaluate behaviors, spend time with people to understand thinking and behaviors
6. Engage, engage, engage, do not just present information in a staff meeting, assign owners to tasks

7. Lead outside the lines; utilize those recognized as informal leaders
8. Inspire others, build pride
9. Leverage formal solutions, reward positive behaviors, provide training that will demonstrate a new functionally or workflow
10. Leverage informal solutions, be aware of those who would undermine the project
11. Assess and adapt, be flexible, measure before and after implementing change (as cited in Aguirre & Alpern, 2014)

It is critical to assess the mood of an organization. An example where the APN PM might encounter issues would be a medical orders implementation or CPOE (computerize provider order entry) in a health system. There are levels of resistance: those who will not learn how to "use a computer" to enter orders so as to threaten "blue flu" during the go live, or those who choose not be involved until the hospital hires scribes to input orders for them. Other successful approaches are to encourage those who are positive about the implementation to be trained as superusers and are the "early adopters" and role models.

As nurses, remember the Kübler-Ross process we all learned with death and dying nursing courses. It has been said that staff go through the same phases with change starting with grief of having to give up or change a comfortable habit they have used. Lewin's three stages of change management methodology was part of a previous course in most master's programs. The stages were unfreezing, change, and refreezing. During the change stage it is important to communicate often, dispel rumors, empower action, and involve people in the processes.

The change management process must include setting up a change control board (CCB) where issues and changes are brought forward at least monthly and even more frequently as the project moves closer to implementation. All of the issues, with action plans to resolve the issues are documented and included in discussion in status meetings. During the meeting the project plan is reviewed and discussed and stakeholders are informed and involved in decision making as indicated.

Lastly, you would also need to add columns for Impact Summary, Change Request Type, Date Identified, Entered By, Actual Resolution Date, and Final Resolution and Rationale, for example, CCB approved.

DELIVERABLES AND CRITICAL SUCCESS FACTORS (CSF)

Deliverables

"Deliverables can be tangible or intangible parts of the development process, and are often specified functions or characteristics of the project" (investopedia.com, 2014). Deliverables were originally identified in the scope document discussed in Chapter 3 and will be the end result or outcome of the project (see Table 4.7).

Critical Success Factors

Rockart (1979) was one of the first to define CSFs as "The limited number of areas in which results, if they are satisfactory, will ensure successful competitive performance for the organization. They are the few key

TABLE 4.7
Sample: Deliverables for XYZ Project

Deliverable	Description	Due Date	Owner
Scope document	Scope	Oct 10, 2016	PM
Charter	Charter	Oct 10 2016	PM
Templates for all project documents	Communication, Risk, RACI plans, all other documents	Oct 10 2016	PM
Budget	Budget	Oct 10, 2016	PM; CFO

CFO, chief financial officer; PM, project manager; RACI, responsible, accountable, consulted, informed.
From Sipes (2014).

TABLE 4.8
Sample: Critical Success Factors (CSF) for XYZ Project by Priority

1. Status reports—appropriate people informed (stakeholders, sponsors; status is documented timely
2. Scope document updated—communicated to all associated with project
3. Budget—project budget is within 5% of original approved budget; projections are reasonable and realistic
4. Charter is updated with all scope changes, approved by key stakeholders and management, and communicated to all
5. Governance—end user buy-in and involvement, timely decision—making, issues and risks resolved timely, project completed on time and on budget

areas where things must go right for the business to flourish. If results in these areas are not adequate, the organization's efforts for the period will be less than desired" (Rockart, 1979, pp. 81–93). CFS are those elements that are critical to a project success (see Table 4.8).

STATUS MEETINGS

Status reports are critical because they provide the timely status of the project at least on a weekly basis. The reports provide updates to the planning and implementation process and establish a pattern of a way to keep everyone informed. These status meetings should be set up from the start of the project. They can be set up in Outlook as recurring over the duration of the project and should include everyone who needs to know and be kept in the loop regarding the status of the project. The meetings occur for 1 hour at least on a weekly basis unless there are issues with the project.

Establish Status Meetings

The status meeting must follow the schedule established and documented in the communication plan. The APN PM must know the status of the project before this meeting. Information is gathered by collecting data from each team member and any others who are involved in the project and assess each task; look for progress, backlogs, or blockages; reflect on key points; and speak to key team members to gain their perspectives. The purpose of the meeting is to keep everyone informed on the status of the project but also to:

- Keep the project moving in the right direction
- Help any new team members assimilate into the team
- Help the team work together—there can be team building activities during the meeting
- Provide time to discuss and address any issues that have arisen between meetings
- Provide time for the PM to coach and mentor the team members
- If there are key issues—that is, the project has yellow or red status—invite key leadership to discuss resolution or how to escalate issues

During the first meeting review the ground rules for meetings such as:

- No cell phones
- Meeting starts on time and ends on time
- Discussions not germane to the topics for the current meeting will be put on the parking lot to be discussed later
- No rabbit trails or war stories
- No side bars
- No "heat-seeking" missiles
- One speaker at a time

Remember that organization, confidence, and respect can be contagious. The PM must be organized and decisive, such as developing a standard status meeting format and meeting agendas. The PM must respect the team members and their time constraints and also be confident in their roles. This sets the stage for the leadership role of the APN as PM and spreads through the team. In order to keep the team focused and moving, remember that even if heavy issues are handled or discussed in the meeting, the PM should always close the meeting on a positive note. Provide positive feedback to the team, encourage and motivate them, and reach out to each member. Applaud the accomplishments to date as well as the ongoing progress. Stress the tremendous teamwork that goes into deliverables coming to fruition. Always leave them with the notion that they are part of a team that is going to complete a successful project by working together and respecting and supporting one another.

Finally, by way of review, the seven steps to a successful meeting include:

1. Plan the meeting
2. Develop an agenda
3. Conduct the meeting
4. Always review the next steps before adjourning the meeting
5. Discuss benefits and concerns the team may have
6. Debrief the meeting—what went well, lessons learned
7. Prepare and distribute minutes within 48 hours of the meeting that includes a plan of action

KICK-OFF MEETING

A kick-off meeting is held when the project has been approved just prior to the next phase—the implementation phase of the project. All project stakeholders, sponsors, administrators, and team members should be included as well as the vendors. The goal of the kick-off meeting is to ensure that everyone is on the same page before the project moves forward to be implemented. It is an opportunity to motivate the team and stakeholders.

Information that will be presented in the meeting includes:

- Goals and objectives of project
- Scope
- Process to request any changes
- Assumptions and constraints
- Risk management plan
- Communication plan
- Each team member's roles and responsibilities
- Schedule and work plan milestones
- Key sponsors and stakeholders

This meeting is also a way to validate the project plan, emphasize the importance of the project, and introduce concepts and team members to leadership and other interested parties. It also sets the expectations and guidelines for the project as well as introduces project sponsors and key stakeholders to the group. It emphasizes the need that everyone on the team be on the same page.

Prepare the PowerPoint Presentation for the Kick-Off Meeting

The first step is to schedule the meeting and include everyone who is affiliated with the project so that they can all hear the same message at the same time. It will be important to provide as many communication methods as possible in case someone can not physically attend the meeting but can access it through conference call or other means, especially if some members are remote.

Next develop the agenda for the meeting and list the invitees. At the onset of the meeting take attendance. Ask the key stakeholders and sponsors for input into the agenda prior to sending it out. Schedule the meeting for 1 hour allowing time at the end for questions and comments, usually 10 minutes. Send the meeting materials out well in advance of the meeting, add it to calendars if Outlook or some other means of scheduling is available, and then send follow-up reminders the day before the meeting. In addition to the earlier list sent, the agenda should include the following:

- Date, time, location including conference call numbers and pass codes
- List of attendees and key contact information for the PM (the PM will have other contact information and should act as the conduit for information)
- Welcome to meeting
- Project plan with itemized list of topics that will be covered and the deliverables
- Review of roles and responsibilities for all team members
- Include a next-steps discussion; finalize any decisions that were not clear if possible
- End with the Q & A session

Send the agenda and other handouts to all attendees including handouts of the PowerPoint presentation. Encourage invitees to bring questions after they have reviewed the project plan and provide comments where relevant.

On the day of the meeting test all communication methods to make sure they have been set up and are functioning properly. Check to make sure the meeting room is set up and equipment is functioning for the PowerPoint presentation. At the start of the meeting, introduce the key stakeholders and sponsors as well as other key invitees—introduce team members. It is always a good idea to invite the stakeholders and/ or sponsors to say a few words but ask them prior to the meeting if they would like to say a few words—do not surprise them during the meeting. These administrators should be positive about the success of the project with an emphasis that this project has priority over other work. The RACI has already been developed; further contract information can be added to that document then provided as a handout during the meeting.

Review all key success factors—these should be key success factors that are specific to the project. It is frustrating when people speak in generalities and do not address the current project. Stay focused and specific. Review the project plan—tasks, responsibilities, milestones, key issues, project dependencies, and risks. This review helps to establish the plan.

Remember to review all plans that have been developed, including the resource-management plan, communication, procurement, and other project documents.

Finally, during the Q & A session, the PM always tries to thoroughly answer all questions and welcomes input. If questions cannot be fully answered, make sure to let the person know when you will get back to him or her with the answer. Typically, the APN PM should have the answers as well as create an atmosphere where team members know the expectations and a culture that respects the work being done as well as demands high-quality work that meets scheduled deadlines.

SUMMARY

This chapter covers some of the most important concepts and principles of project management as the APN as PM begins to apply the concepts to a project. The APN PM also has learned to develop new tools that will be needed to closely track the progress of the project. Resource management is critical to the success of a project. Having a schedule is critical to successful resource management. Therefore, it is important to understand how to create a schedule. One tool that can be used is a network diagram. The project's activities are assigned to the people who will be doing the work. They build duration estimates for the activities. The most accurate estimates are built from previous experience with similar projects. This allows you to determine a project's scheduled completion time, the slack or float of project activities, and the critical path of your project.

REFERENCES

Activity sequencing and network diagrams. (2014). Retrieved from https://www .e-education.psu.edu/geog584/l5_p4.html

Aguirre, D., & Alpern, M. (2014). *10 Principles of leading change management; time-honored tools and techniques*. Retrieved from www.strategy-business.com

Aguirre, D., & Rutger, V. P. (2013). *Culture and change management survey.* Retrieved November, 2014, from www.strategy-business.com

Baker, S. (2013). *Critical path method (CPM)*. Retrieved from https://h5pm.sph .www.sc.edu/courses/J716/CPM/CPM.html

Change management log template. (2010). Retrieved from http://www2a.cdc .gov/cdcup/library/other/help/html

Communications management plan (CMP). (2014). CDC United States Department of Health and Human Services. www.hhs.gov

Create a network diagram—office support. (2014). Retrieved from office.microsoft/create-a-network-diagram. https://support.office.com/...3e8cc62-27c5

Critical path method. (2014). Summer, 2014/Issue 75; Retrieved from www .tutorialspoint.com/managementconcepts/criticalpathmethod

Critical path method and PERT. (2014). Retrieved from http://www.mindtools .com/critpath.html

Critical Success Factors. (2014). Identifying the things that really matter for success. http://www.washington.edu/research/rapid/resources/toolsTem plate/art_success_factors.pdf

Definition of activity in a box, network diagram. (2014). Retrieved from www. businessdictionary.com/definition/activity-network-diagram

Deliverables defined. (2014). Retrieved from www.investopedia.com/terms/d/ deliverables.asp

How to customize the network diagram; view in Microsoft Project. (2014). Retrieved from www.projectknowledge.net

Identification of the critical path. (2014). Retrieved from www.tutorialspoint.com

Morris, R. (2014). *The network diagram*. Retrieved from www.netplaces.com/ project-management

Nishadha. (2012). *Importance of critical path method in project planning*. Retrieved from http://creately.com

Rockart J. (1979). Chief executives define their own data needs. *Harvard Business Review 57*(2), 81-93.

ADDITIONAL READING

Adamm, J. J. (2014). Review of the book Project management in health and community services: Getting ideas to work (2nd ed.) *Australian Journal of Primary Health, 20*(1), 122.

Communication: The message is clear; White Paper. Newtown Square, PA: PMI. http://www.pmi.org

Covey, F. (2012). Franklin Covey Co. launches project management essentials for the unofficial PM: anyone can be a successful project manager. *Business Wire*. Retrieved from investor.franklincovey.com

Heldman, K. (2013). *PMP: Project management professional*. New York, NY: Wiley.

Ho, J. (2010). Project management in health informatics. *Studies in Health Technology & Informatics, 151*, 413-424.

CHAPTER 5

Implementation/Execution—Phase 3

LEARNING OBJECTIVES

Upon completion of this chapter, the reader will be able to:

1. Define the implementation phase
2. Discuss three tasks to be accomplished during the implementation phase
3. Discuss the value of a change management plan
4. Discuss three steps to developing the change management plan
5. Discuss why it is important to engage stakeholders
6. Discuss why it is important to define and monitor critical success factors (CSF)

OUTLINE

- Key Terms
- Overview of Project Implementation
- Implementing Project Management Plans
- Implementation Checklist
- Managing Project Teams: Leadership Skills
- Managing Project Stakeholders
- Status Meetings
- Change Management in the Implementation Phase
- Minimizing Scope Changes
- Communication Plan in the Implementation Phase
- Testing
- Quality Control

KEY TERMS

Execute
Implementation
Key performance indicator (KPI)
Metrics
Lewin's change theory

Phases/Steps of project
management
Stakeholders
Testing

The next step in project management is the implementation, which corresponds to the implementation phase of the nursing process. Project implementation "requires that everyone involved, including the members of the unit staff understand the goal, expectations, and timeline. A well-run project allows all participants to be able to instantly access the data. Success depends on every team member being a part of the implementation process in ways that are vital and change oriented. Every team member is responsible for investigating why mistakes made will contribute to the process change" (Overgaard, 2010, p. 53)

Nursing and project management go well together and overlap in many processes. As discussed earlier, project management includes: project initiation, planning, implementation, monitoring, and closing. "Originally conceived as a tool to ensure that projects using many disciplines would be correctly budgeted and completed within a scheduled time frame, project management has become useful in a variety of settings from writing a book to building a skyscraper. The use of the systematic steps in project management can eliminate costly mistakes, increase quality, and save time" (Project Planning, Delivery, and Controls, 2014). As discussed in Chapter 2, correlations to the nursing process were demonstrated and may help the nurse manager understand how using a systematic process to complete a project is beneficial.

In this step, phase 3 of project management, the project will be implemented or executed as some organizations refer to this. You will begin to apply the tools that were discussed and developed in the previous phases. The project activities such as applying the concepts of monitor and control will help you step into the role of project manager (PM). In this phase of project management, tool implementation developed in the previous phases—design and planning—will be implemented.

OVERVIEW OF PROJECT IMPLEMENTATION

In the previous phases you learned that there are five standard phases to a project: design/initiation, planning, implementation/execution, monitor and control, and closing the project where evaluation and lessons learned are conducted. Some organizations have combined steps and refer to only four steps in the process, while others may break the steps out further and refer to six steps in the project management process. Whichever process best fits the project or activity it is important to remember that you may use all of the steps or only a few. It is important to remember, too, that a "project" is only a temporary activity such as planning a wedding or developing a project for a graduate practicum, just as the steps in developing a patient care plan can be a temporary activity.

Five Standard Project Management Phases: Similar to the Nursing Process

The five standard project management phases or stages are very similar to the nursing processes and are described here.

Design/Initiation

The design/initiation process establishes the feasibility and goals of the project. It is during this phase that the project is authorized. Many times there is some confusion regarding the project management terminology that is used by an organization. Frequently both terms are used—design and initiation—as the first phase where the project starts to come together with thoughts and ideas of what should happen in the project. In this first phase, the project charter and scope documents are developed; these documents help provide direction to the project.

Planning

The project plan addresses the triple constraints of cost, quality, and schedule. This is the phase where activities are defined or the work related to the project and a schedule are developed for the project. The project plan should include the goals, deliverables, schedule, communication strategy, risk management, work breakdown structure (WBS), network diagram, budget, and a human resources plan. Stakeholders should also be identified at this point. The work is now planned and will be implemented as the tools that were developed in this second phase of the project management are applied. The phase ends with the kick-off meeting.

Implementation/Execution

Here again, many times different terminology is used to mean the same thing depending on the organization. More frequently today, the term project implementation is used to mean this is the third phase of project management—where implementation of all of the tools happens, including adding resources team members, and the applications that were previously tested and built. This is when the plan that was developed in previous phases of project management is implemented where the content from both the scope and charter documents, as well as all of the tools such as the risk, change management, communication and other documents, are implemented. Status meetings will be established as part of the communication plan. A human resources plan will be implemented that includes how the team will develop and be nurtured, as well as specific assignments that will need to be completed. The communication plan will be finalized for the stakeholders and the risk management plan will be implemented.

Monitor and Control

The monitor and control processes are ongoing throughout the entire project; any issues need to be quickly addressed. Change requests will be monitored very closely—there may even be denial of changes or changes may need to be moved to a different time or phase for implementation—depending on the total project impact. This is when the status of the project is monitored in relation to the schedule. A key question to ask is, "Are the steps when controlling and monitoring the schedule delineated to indicate on time, at or under budget, and the production of quality products?"

Closing and Evaluation

Typically, the last phase of project management is closing and evaluation of the project. It entails resolving any issues and completion of all necessary final documents and reports for terminating the project. The team will debrief and compile useful information, such as lessons learned concerning the completed project, for current and future reference of what worked well and what would need improvement before utilizing again. The information will then be presented to the stakeholders in a final PowerPoint presentation where the PM will receive final verification and sign-off from leadership.

IMPLEMENTING PROJECT MANAGEMENT PLANS

Primary Objectives

The main objective as the project is implemented is to apply the concepts, tools, and methods discussed in the previous chapters that will support the ongoing management of the project. The outcome of the project will be a deliverable that meets the requirements of the organization. The primary objectives when implementing a project are:

- To apply a standardized method and steps in an organized way so that creation of the project "deliverable" is completed in an orderly way and that steps or important elements of the project are not overlooked. It is very important to remember that if you do not have the time to do it right the first time, when would you find time and money to do it over? The art of being consistent is also very important to team members as it provides stability rather than constant change.
- It is important to be as transparent as possible with the team members and stakeholders so they can anticipate the next steps in the project development.

- Learn to be a good decision maker—be timely and goal orientated, consult team and stakeholders when necessary. Provide project updates daily, weekly, whatever process was established as you develop the project plan. If there are requests for more information, revise the communication plan.
- Remember to monitor the constraints that have been identified as critical to the project, which includes, but are not limited to, being on budget and on time when delivering the business objectives of the project.
- If resources do not have a specific commitment to this project, monitor them closely as they may be shared with other projects or have other time commitments.

Implementing/Executing the Project

Review the implementation/execution phase with team and stakeholders. Make sure that there is a thorough understanding of the plan by all so it can be monitored to keep the project and everyone moving in the right direction. Remember to build and nurture the teams as well as to manage the project and communicate, communicate, communicate.

IMPLEMENTATION CHECKLIST

The project management methodology has been discussed and the tools needed to monitor and control the implementation were developed in phase 2–planning step. The next step is to apply both the processes and tools. The main components of implementation include those found in Table 5.1.

It is best to keep a copy of the checklist available to check off tasks in progress and/or completed at least on a weekly basis.

Apply Toolkit Developed During Design and Planning Phases to Maintain Updated Project Plan

The main objective is to review the work plan on a regular basis to determine how the project is progressing in terms of schedule, budget, scope, risks, and issues. Basic objectives to accomplish this are to monitor the

TABLE 5.1
Implementation Checklist

Steps	Activity	Responsibility	Due Date
1	Maintain updated project plan and evaluation	Project manager	
2	Monitor tasks and document next steps	Project manager	
3	Manage issues and escalate as necessary	Project manager; project team, stakeholders	
4	Manage and report risks	Project manager; project team, stakeholders	
5	Develop CPM and monitor	Project manger	
6	Manage budget	Project manager; stakeholders	
7	Manage project communications and presentations	Project manager; project team	
8	Mange meetings—team, stakeholders, other executives	Project manager; project team, stakeholders	
9	Manage and create timely status reports	Project manager	
10	Document, document, document	Project manager; project team	
11	Evaluate need for education and training	Project manager; project team	

CPM, critical path method.
From Sipes (2014).

progress from the beginning of the project to avoid surprises. Revise the plan for accuracy; if changes are required they will need to go to the change control board (CCB) that has been established. Has new work been identified that may have been overlooked? Review the project milestones—are they on schedule? Are they being impacted by other tasks?

Other activities to monitor include a review of activities that have been completed and update the plan to reflect this. Determine what resources were used and if they impacted the current plan in any way. Review the plan to assess if any tasks have been delayed and determine the cause as well as other tasks that might be impacted.

As the plan is updated, review the due dates again to make sure the project is on time, conduct a critical path using the critical path method (CPM) example discussed in the planning phase. Work with team members and stakeholders to determine ways to accelerate tasks to get back on track. As the plan is updated, it is important to include the team members, to remain transparent, and include all communication with the team and other stakeholders. Conduct a review of all dates, status, description of the tasks and resolution of issues and the owner. Review next steps to make sure they are accurate. Document any changes required, document and also send to the CCB for review and sign-off if needed. Identify and review with the team any work that is not currently in the plan. Review if and how it will impact the project, that is, if you delay the project by days or weeks, will it impact another task or subtask? Any delay in a milestone will need to be evaluated by leadership, executives and stakeholders to determine the impact on the entire project. An evaluation of the project can be crashed or pushed to meet deadlines will be reviewed and decisions made.

In summary, critical success factors (CSF) to implementing a project include monitoring that all tasks are completed effectively, on time, and within budget. Monitoring that all team members maintain responsibility for the tasks assigned to them and that there are not task delays due to lack of task completion is also critical. Finally, monitoring that all risks have been identified and mitigated and that there are no remaining tasks that are not resolvable is another CSF. In this phase—implementation— is where the toolkit and documents will be applied as well as the concepts previously created. Important to close monitoring and control of the project will be the potential need to revise and update any tools and documents then reapply them to the project.

MANAGING PROJECT TEAMS: LEADERSHIP SKILLS

You may not assume the role of PM with a project team working with you, depending on the project you are working on. Or you may be asked to assume one of the project management roles as part of the graduate practicum experience. One important aspect of management is to understand the difference between a manager and a leader. You will have an opportunity, or may have had in the past, to research and study a number of leadership theories, such as transformational leadership, and how to apply them, but that is not the purpose here. The purpose is to reflect on what you do as a manager and how that applies to what you do as you develop as a leader.

Nurses have assumed management roles for many decades—this is not a new concept. Historically, Florence Nightingale was both a manager and a leader (Gardner, 1986; Huxley, 1975). She managed, changed, and revolutionized the health system in the British military in the mid-19th century. You may become or are familiar with many leadership theories that define the skills used and that are inherent to good leaders.

You may have had a chance to shadow a mentor or other manager during a practicum experience. Have you had a chance to reflect on how management and leadership overlap? As an advance practice nurse, you will now be expected to assume more leadership roles. Gardner's work is considered foundational as he has conducted a number of research studies on leadership. According to Gardner (1993; Gardner & Avolio, 1998), leadership and management overlap in many ways and "most managers exhibit some leadership skills, and most leaders ... find themselves managing" (pp. 6, 7). Leadership and management are not the same things, but they overlap. It makes sense to include the specifics of managing in the list of tasks leaders perform (see Table 5.2).

As you work with others on your project team think about how what you are doing fits as a manager or leader. As a new manager you have learned a number of skills in the graduate program. You have had the opportunity to apply those skills and experience the outcomes of the skills and tasks you have completed as you become more skilled as a PM (see Box 5.1).

Other qualities are important as a leader and manager, which also can be defined as project management attributes. These include the importance of motivating team members, planning and priority setting, organizing,

TABLE 5.2
Overlap Between Leaders and Managers

Leaders	Managers
Set goals	Set goals
Plan	Plan
Set priorities	Set priorities
Keep system functioning by setting agendas	Keep system functioning by setting agendas
Make decisions	Make decisions

Adapted by Sipes (2014) from Gardner (1993).

BOX 5.1 REFLECTION

But how are the functional activities you do as a PM different because you also have a theatrical background and deeper learning and other qualities you bring as a nurse leader to your project team? Reflect on the opportunities you have had to interact and empower different team members, your mentor, and even other leaders. What are some key attributes you will take from these experiences? Reflect on what you will and will not do in the future as you incorporate the concepts of project management into your role and define the type of leader you are or want to be.

---

allocating resources, agenda setting, and decision making. Do these attributes sound like those discussed previously as project management skills?

As Gardner noted, leadership skills include:

- Motivating: Effective leaders tap those that serve the purposes of collective action in pursuit of shared goals. They accomplish the alignment of individual and group goals. ... They create a climate in which there is pride in making significant contributions to shared goals.
- Managing: ... Leadership and management are not the same thing, but they overlap. It makes sense to include managing in the list of tasks leaders perform.
  - Someone has to plan ... and set priorities
  - Someone has to ... design the structures and processes through which substantial endeavors get accomplished over time
  - Someone has to keep the system functioning ... mobilizing and ... allocating resources; ... directing, delegating and coordinating; ... reporting, evaluating and holding accountable
  - Someone has to ... set agendas and make decisions (1993, p. 6)

It is important to reflect on pressures you may encounter as a "leader." According to Gardner et al. (2005), "we are told that people look for organizational leaders of character and integrity to provide direction and help them find meaning in their work" (p. 344).

MANAGING PROJECT STAKEHOLDERS

Stakeholders who were identified in the design phase by definition have a vested interest in the project and need to be kept informed of the project status. They need to be identified and the buy-in obtained early on and maintained throughout the project. It is important to respect their time so it will be important to prepare a succinct status report for stakeholders. The resources that have an interest in the project were identified earlier—now you will need to prepare a status report for this phase of the project for them.

Stakeholder Presentations

You will need to communicate to determine what your stockholders expect in the way of status reports, be it weekly, bi-weekly or only on a monthly basis. It will be important to obtain a signature/sign-off for each report presented. The reports must be succinct and to the point, so prepare only key points. In the report include:

- An introduction of key stakeholders
- Project objectives
- Project issues
- Project barriers
- Next steps with owners
- Due dates

The goal of the stakeholder reports is to get approval and acceptance for the progress made on the project and to keep them informed of all steps in the project progress. It is important to remember, these are very important people who have an interest in and support for the project. If this is a graduate practicum project for both master's and DNP programs, and you are working with your mentor, this group helped to identify the project deliverables as well as provide funding for the project. A stakeholder can also be an end user who had input into how the project should be designed and then implemented. If there are a number of end users, it is best to have one or two representatives of the group in attendance at these presentations. If there are too many attendees with opposing views of how the project is to be implemented, it can delay the project further and prevent closing of the project in a timely manner.

The one thing to remember is that change is constant. The monitor and control documents and examples are discussed in Chapter 6. They should be used throughout the project to identify changes that need to be made then presented to the CCB. By now you have discovered how many different processes must be constantly monitored and controlled. Good project management also depends on the project team and performance against the constraints of time, cost, and scope.

Key ongoing tasks that should be monitored for possible revisions and updates include:

- Project plan
- Project objectives
- Project milestones and timeline
- Project performance metrics
- Project issues, risks
- Project change control
- Project team performance

Reflect on the key tasks you should be monitoring and some reasons why projects fail. Do you see the potential correlation between the two? What process will you use to do this? How will you document the process? Where will you present the information?

STATUS MEETINGS

Status meetings and status reports were discussed in Chapter 4. One of the most important tasks a PM must undertake is to communicate effectively with all team members and leadership. One critical component is to plan and hold effective and productive meetings as previously discussed. An effective and productive meeting can also enhance decision making for the project. It is important to set goals and objectives for the meeting to provide a framework for effective decision making. This is now where the application of what was previously planned is implemented. There are seven key steps to conducting an effective meeting. See Table 5.3 for content needed in status reports. By way of review, these are:

1. Plan the meeting
2. Always have an agenda; create the agenda with goals, objectives, and times; distribute before the meeting

TABLE 5.3
Weekly Project Status Report

Project Name:	**Week Ending:**
Project ID:	**Project Manager:**
Description of Project:	**Project Start Date:**
Project End Date:	**% Complete**
Project Issues:	**Causes:**
Project Risks:	**Proposed Mitigation:**

Project Is On Time, On Budget, Within Scope
Green (OK)   Yellow (In trouble—Watch)   Red (In danger—Escalate)
Sign-off: Project Manager: Stakeholder: CEO/Other Leadership:

From Sipes (2014).

3. Conduct the meeting; start and stop on time; review ground rules; no rabbit trails; document conversations/minutes; document participants

4. Review next steps; assign owners to different tasks and document with due dates

5. Document benefits and concerns (B & Cs); there are no wrong answers

6. Summarize—what went well, what could have gone better, lessons learned

7. Write up, record decisions, next meeting date, and distribute minutes within 48 hours of meeting; one-page summary with attachments if necessary

CSF for any meeting should include an informed leadership of issues and progress. Team members are kept up to date on project activities, status, and the decision-making process. Finally, decisions regarding any changes are made within the critical timeframes defined.

CHANGE MANAGEMENT IN THE IMPLEMENTATION PHASE

"Sometimes the problem is not outright conflict but an unwillingness to cooperate. One of the gravest problems George Washington faced as a general was that the former colonies, though they had no doubt they were all on the same side, were not always sure they wanted to cooperate" (Gardner, 1993, p. 7).

In the implementation phase is it important to understand the processes and rationale behind change theory and why an understanding of what happens is important to the changes that will occur during implementation. If you are implementing a project for a graduate practicum as an advanced practice nurse (APN), the one thing you are learning as you progress through the practicum is that change is constant. Monitor and control documents will be developed and will be used to identify changes that needs to be made and presented to the CCB.

Ten principles for changes were discussed in Chapter 4, which should help understanding. There was also an example of a change management log. Change management theories will also help to better understand how to apply change in nursing practice, dealing with how nurses use change, information, and knowledge to make sound practice judgments. Just as nursing science deals with nursing and the nursing process, project management specifically addresses how to integrate and use project management process and tools to enhance management of patient care issues. Understanding change by exploring change theory and diffusion of innovation theory helps to explain behaviors that may be seen before changes occur. By helping those involved in the change will provide for the betterment of patient care outcomes. Exploring change theory and how it might apply to the team and others involved in change is important.

Diffusion of Innovation Theory

The two theories important to explore are diffusion of innovation theory and change theory. The diffusion of innovation theory explores those who lead opinions, those who follow, and how the media can influence the opinion leaders as well as the opinion followers. The theory describes the process that people go through to adopt something new, such as a product, idea, practice, philosophy, or other theory. The theory is very important in project management because new things are introduced, and this theory helps understanding the diffusion or process through which the innovation is or is not adopted (see Box 5.2).

BOX 5.2 REFLECTION—DIFFUSION OF INNOVATION AND
CHANGE THEORIES

- When you read Kaminski's (2011) diffusion of innovation arti-
  cle on change, reflect on a change that you experienced in relation to some point in the project management process up to
  this point. As you learned new ideas, how did that occur? Can
  you relate it to the diffusion of innovation theory?
- Change theory is another important theory by Lewin. Change
  theory describes a three-phase process in which we open our
  minds, deal with the change, and adopt the change. It is important to understand the dynamics when dealing with change
  and expecting others to deal with change also. Think about
  different reactions to the change. Can you trace the phases as
  described by Lewin?

Lewin's Change Theory

Some rules for effective management of change. Managing organizational change will be more successful if applying these simple
principles. Achieving personal change will be more successful too
when using the same approach where relevant. Change management
entails thoughtful planning and sensitive implementation and, above
all, consultation with, and involvement of, the people affected by the
changes.

If change is forced on people, normally problems arise. Change must
be realistic, achievable, and measurable. These aspects are especially
relevant to managing personal change. Before starting organizational
change ask "What do we want to achieve with this change, why, and
how will we know that the change has been achieved? Who is affected
by this change, and how will they react to it? How much of this change
can be achieved ourselves, and what parts of the change need help?"
These aspects also relate strongly to the management of personal as well
as organizational change.

TABLE 5.4
Change Request Form

Identification of Change	Data
Change Request	Change request #; date received; date revised; project #, name, requester name, department
Requestor Information	Describe change, reason, priority;
Change Information	Impact on stakeholders, organization
Status Information	Next Steps: owner, date, decision, due date
CCB Approvals	Signatures

CCB, change control board.
From Sipes (2014).

In summary, theoretical applications in nursing as an APN are critical to the success of practical application and the ability to implement potent systems that enhance patient care. Think about the theories that are used in practice and the theories that you have begun to use during this graduate practicum journey.

Change Management Tracking Tool

The concept of a change management board has been discussed several times. Most organizations have a CCB or change management team that usually meets at least once a month 3 months before a project is implemented then bi-weekly 1 to 3 months before implementation/go-live, as more issues arise at that time. Principles of control for project change should include the appropriate stakeholders who are or might be involved in the evaluation and approval process with all proposed scope changes documented to be evaluated and approved before they are implemented. Any and all change requests are assessed for impact on other components of the project and other projects currently in development. Project changes are communicated to both team members and any other stakeholders for evaluation and feedback as well as approval before progressing further.

MINIMIZING SCOPE CHANGES

Minimizing scope change must be continually assessed in order to prevent scope creep.

Reasons for Unplanned Scope Changes

To better understand what might cause changes in your scope plan you need to understand the potential reasons that might cause the project to change. Some of these reasons might be related to:

- A shift in business focus
- Change in timeline
- Change in budget and funding sources
- Change in key sponsor, stakeholder, and other leadership commitment
- Change in technology requirements, upgrades, new vendor products
- Unclear definition of overall project requirements and support where requirements are not aligned with overall organizational scope

All of the areas listed here need to be fully evaluated by the PM and project team and reported to stakeholders and leadership to define and develop a plan for mitigation of the changes.

COMMUNICATION PLAN IN THE IMPLEMENTATION PHASE

Types of Communication

Communication as a skill was discussed in Chapter 4. During the implementation phase, a communication plan will need to be developed and communicated to the project team and all invested in the project. When developing the communication plan for the project and team, it is important to consider different types or ways of communicating effectively. It is important to remember that people have different learning styles; therefore, creating a communication style that fits the different learning styles will go a long way to effective communication. A summary of the types of communication are listed in Table 5.5.

Communication Mistakes

Being a good communicator takes skill, practice and continual effort. Good communication is difficult and is an art. Have you ever sent off a

TABLE 5.5
Communication Plan

Type of Information	Participants	Purpose	Frequency	Transmittal	Prepared by
Status Meetings	Project team sponsor	Report project status, including significant accomplishments, issues, and costs	Distributed prior to the scheduled meeting	E-mail Meeting	Project manager
Change Requests	Program staff Project sponsor Project manager	Communicate, receive approval and document status of all change requests	As needed	E-mail Meeting	Project manager
Project Plan	Project team	To articulate project background, scope, roles/responsibilities, risk, deliverables, schedule, staffing, communication, and close-out	At project start-up	E-mail	Project manager
Kick-Off Meeting	Project team	The kick-off meeting is used to clarify goals and objectives, individual roles and responsibilities, interdependencies	Once at project start-up	Meeting	Project manager Meeting
Weekly Status Meeting	Project team	Discuss status, issues and concerns related to the project	Weekly	Oral presentation Discussions	Project manager

Adapted from CA Dept. of Trans (2014).

message or written a document that has numerous typos and spelling errors? Or have you read a document or email from someone else full of errors? What was your impression of that person? Have you ever attended a meeting where there was no direction or agenda? How did that make you feel? Disorganized?

Another frequently cited error is delivering bad news via e-mail, which should really be done in a personal communication, or, even worse, by forwarding others' e-mails that were not intended for others to see, potentially violating privacy.

A mistake new PMs frequently make is to assume everyone under-stands exactly what is being said. In this case it is important to ask for questions and use multiple approaches to getting your message out. Never assume that your messages are always understood. Always have an open mind to other effective ways of completing a task or suggestion.

TESTING

One of the most important functions a PM can oversee and manage is that of testing of the deliverable has been developed. Unfortunately, when there is a time crunch on a project, testing is the one function that is cut back or eliminated. It is also a reason the project might fail. You may have experienced this or remember the issues with the health care system or a smaller project roll-out.

Why Is Testing Important?

This concept is so important it is discussed again in Chapter 6. As a review, CNN News reported, "An internal government memo written just days before the start of open enrollment for Obamacare warned of a 'high' security risk because of a lack of testing of the HealthCare.gov website." Additional comments from CNN, "officials of companies hired to create the HealthCare.gov website cited a lack of testing on the full system and last-minute changes by the federal agency overseeing the online enrollment system."

Testing is typically broken down into five phases:

1. Individual programming modules
2. Integration
3. Volume
4. System as a whole
5. Acceptance or beta testing

Systems are designed by application or module; each module or application is first tested individually. Depending on the testing process, the individual applications or modules are gradually integrated then tested. Finally, all of the applications that have been tested and passed are moved into the entire system where it is then tested as a whole.

Acceptance or beta testing is the final phase before implementation of a system and refers to whole system testing, corrections made, with the final step as implementation. You may be involved or have an opportunity to view the testing processes that will provide valuable information and insight into the project management process and lead to understanding of how critical the testing phase is.

You may also hear the term usability testing. The key principles of usability are simplicity, naturalness, consistency, minimizing cognitive load, efficient interactions, forgiveness and feedback, effective use of language, effective information presentation, and preservation of context (HIMSS, 2009). It is important to understand how this fits with testing as these are many of the elements incorporated into test scripts that are used by testers. A Healthcare Information Management Systems Society (HIMSS) survey (2009) reports that one reason electronic medical record (EMR) adoption and implementation rates have been very slow is due to lack of efficiency and usability of current systems.

QUALITY CONTROL

Key Performance Indicators

You frequently hear about key performance indicators (KPIs), but what is a KPI? A KPI is a business metric used to evaluate factors that are crucial to the success of an organization (http://searchcrm.techtarget.com). When selecting a KPI, it is important to keep it simple with a limited number of KPIs, so that the target can be attained. It also needs to meet the organization's missions and goals. For example, leadership will meet to determine these and invite suggestions from other leaders and managers with the ultimate goal of having three or four KPIs that support the organizational goals and mission. KPIs predict performance and are specifically linked to a strategic objective that help an organization translate organizational strategy execution into quantifiable terms.

Examples might be increased patient satisfaction, decreased number of patients left-without-being-seen (LWBS), minutes until patients are seen in the emergency department, reduced employee turnover by XXX per year if it tracks to the mission statement and goals. Whichever

KPIs are selected, they must be measureable and quantifiable and reflect the organization's success. Each KPI must have a target including a due date, the same requirements when developing project objectives (http://management.about.com).

Metrics

According to Becher (2006), "all KPIs are metrics, but not all metrics are KPIs. An organization may have many metrics, but few KPIs" (2006, p. 14). Metrics can represent anything, but KPIs are said to matter most. KPIs should also be tied to an objective, such as "this will be due on XXX" or "this rate will be reduced by XXX%," which is defined by specific objectives that answer the five "Ws" and "H" (Sipes, 2014)—the who, what, where, when, why, and how?

So when is a metric a KPI? KPIs are metrics that meet the five "W" criteria.

The criteria, the five Ws, should be used in evaluating whether a metric meets KPI status and help ensure focus on the measures that truly matter to the success of the organization.

SUMMARY

The chapter provides the tools and concepts used in the implementation phase, the third phase of project management. In this phase tools that were developed in the design and planning phases are implemented and processes are tracked, monitored, and controlled. Leadership skills are discussed as well as change management theories with suggestions on how to manage change and different behaviors that might be seen during this phase. Finally, quality control measures and processes such as determining KPIs and metrics are defined and suggestions for what and how they might be used are provided.

REFERENCES

Becher, J. (2006). Mitigating metrics madness: How to tell KPIs from mere metrics. *19*(4). Retrieved from www.cutter.com

California Department of Transportation. (2014). *Communication plan*. Retrieved from www.dot.ca.gov

Gardner, J. W. (1993). *On leadership*. New York, NY: The Free Press. Retrieved from www.altfeldinc.com/pdfs/JohnWGardner.pdf

Gardner, W. L., & Avolio, B. J. (1998). The charismatic relationship: A dramaturgical perspective. *Academy of Management Review, 23*, 32–58.

Gardner, W. L., Avolio, B. J., Luthans, F., May, D. R., & Walumba, F. O. (2005). Can you see the real me? A self-based model of authentic leader and follower development. *The Leadership Quarterly. 16*(3), 343–372.

Healthcare Information Management Systems Society (HIMSS). (2009). A call for action: Enabling healthcare reform using information technology. Retrieved from www.himss.org/2009calltoaction

HealthCare.gov. http://www.networkworld.com/article/2171176/data-center/contractors—more-testing-of healthcare-gov-was-needed.html

Huxley, E.J. (1975). *Florence Nightingale*. New York, NY: Putnam.

Kaminski, J. (2011a). Theory applied to informatics: Lewin's change theory. [Editorial]. *CJNI: Canadian Journal of Nursing Informatics, 6*(1). Retrieved from http://cjni.net/journal/?p=1210

Kaminski, J. (2011b). Theory in Nursing Informatics Column: Diffusion of innovation theory. *CJNI: Canadian Journal of Nursing Informatics, 6*(2). Retrieved from http://cjni.net/journal/?p=1444

National Institute of Building Sciences. (2014). *Project planning, delivery, and controls*. Retrieved from http://www.wbdg.org/project/pm.php#mr

Overgaard, P. (2010). Get the keys to successful project management, *Nursing Management, 41*(6), 53–54. doi:10.1097/01.NUMA.0000381744.25529.e8

Project planning, delivery, and controls. (2014). https://www.wbdg.org/project. *11*(7) p. 1. Author

CHAPTER 6

Monitoring and Controlling the Project—Phase 4

LEARNING OBJECTIVES

Upon completion of this chapter, the reader will be able to:

1. Define three components of the monitor and control phase
2. Discuss three tasks to be accomplished during the monitor and control phase
3. Discuss the value of monitoring and controlling a project
4. Discuss when the monitor and control functions should be implemented
5. Discuss three reasons projects fail
6. Discuss the 80/20 rule
7. Discuss one method to monitor the quality of a project

OUTLINE

- Key Terms
- Overview of Monitoring and Controlling a Project
- Implementation of the Monitor and Control Plan
- Benefits and Process of Monitoring
- Benefits and Process of Change Control
- Quality Control—Root Cause Analysis
- Testing

KEY TERMS

80/20 rule
Critical success factors (CSF)
Deming's plan, do, check, act
   (PDCA) cycle

Milestones
Pareto principle
Root cause analysis

The monitor and control process is about managing the juggling act that the project manager (PM) must master during the project implementation process. In the previous chapter, the discussion centered on how to implement a project when using different processes and tools. This chapter covers the "what, why, and how" to conduct the ongoing project management.

With implementation comes the monitoring and controlling that must occur throughout a project. Monitoring and controlling project processes makes sure that the project team is completing its work correctly and according to the project plan. It might feel like trying to manage the universe at times: time, money, teams, product, communication, quality, and the list go on. All of these elements must be monitored and controlled in order to have a successful project. This is where the PM must keep everything flowing and truly manage scope, time, and cost. Using the tools that were developed in the design and planning phases will provide the guidelines needed to manage the project.

Finally, as you continue to manage the project, there is a need to continually evaluate the project progress against the original goals and objectives you initially developed for this project, as well as the mission statement, timeline, and project plan.

OVERVIEW OF MONITORING AND CONTROLLING A PROJECT

Standard Processes

The monitor and control process of a project requires frequent checking to make sure all tasks are applied in a standardized way, that there is frequent communication of the project status, that there are effective decisions made toward achieving the goals, and that the deliverables identified in the scope meet the due dates and meet quality standards. Finally, it is important to determine that resources continually meet the requirements for completing the project in a standardized way.

IMPLEMENTATION OF THE MONITOR AND CONTROL PLAN

Primary Objective

Key to monitoring the project at this phase is to review the project plan on a regular basis—at least weekly if not more frequently—to determine how the project is moving forward in terms of time, due dates, budget, scope, issues, and risks.

Other objectives that will greatly impact the project require that the project be monitored from the very beginning of implementation to avoid surprises. If there are problems, evaluate and revise the plan to make sure the activity can be monitored and tracked. Be sure that all new work not currently in the project plan has been identified and assigned an owner. Evaluate the project milestones and due dates to determine if dates are being met. If there is an issue, consider conducting a critical path analysis and/or ways to crash the project. These processes were discussed in Chapter 4.

Activities

All activities should be closely monitored and included on the timeline as well as identification of the activities that were previously completed so that the project plan can be updated and resources reassigned if necessary. Always track and report the percent complete in the weekly status reports, especially the information that goes to the leadership and stakeholders. The weekly status report tool is available in Chapter 5. Closely review all activities to make sure that all dependencies are completed prior to the activity being sure to indicate what those are and how they might impact other activities. After completing this assessment be sure to update the project plan and send the new, updated copies to all stakeholders.

If the plan needs to be revised, obtain the needed information requesting feedback from every team member, then hold a status meeting so that all team members can determine if and how changes might impact their tasks. Include all team members in the decisions and determination of next steps as well as update due dates if indicated. Finally, communicate, communicate, and communicate to set expectations for all involved in the project including the stakeholders and leadership. Also document the objectives, expectations, problems, milestones, (CSF) and critical success factors.

New Work

If new work has been identified during the monitoring and controlling process, pull the team together and have everyone participate to determine who "owns" the new work, the due dates, and if it really is part of another task or should be moved to the next phase. Review to understand if the new work is associated with a milestone. If not, establish one and document it in the work plan. You will find budget tracking tools, as well as application and processes used, in Chapter 4.

Budget

During implementation, it is necessary to track the budget very closely to determine how much of the budget has actually been used based on tasks completed and then determine how much money is left as you ask "Is the project on budget?" Also review to determine where future large expenses might occur so that these can be planned accordingly. It is important to get weekly reports back from team members during the status meetings to determine how much work remains.

BENEFITS AND PROCESS OF MONITORING

Why Projects Fail

As previously discussed, there are many different processes that must constantly be monitored and controlled. Good project management also depends on the project team and their performance against the constraints—time, cost, quality, risks, and scope. It is important to reflect on how well the process is going with frequent discussions of how to do things a bit differently going forward if problems arise. There are many reasons why projects might fail. Here are a few key reasons to keep in mind:

- Someone on the team wanted to help out an end user by just "tweaking" an application and thought there would be no impact on the system, but in fact took the system down leading to delays and cost overruns.
- Scope creep—doing "favors" for end users or stakeholders, adding additional tasks that are outside of the budget
- Lack of good communication with the team and among leadership. For example, the stakeholder thought the project was to solve problem XXX when the direction of the project is going YYY.

One way to help mitigate the risk of failure is to constantly reconfirm any plan against the project plan, objectives, the scope, and charter documents. Good, ongoing communication is critical with not only the project team but with leadership and stakeholders who have an interest in and are committed to this project.

Key ongoing tasks that should be monitored, if not daily at least three to four times a week, include:

- Project plan
- Project objectives
- Project milestones and timeline
- Project performance metrics
- Project issues, risks
- Project change control
- Project team performance

When the monitor and control documents were created then applied to the project, were there questions that were overlooked or not considered such as:

- Who will be accountable, in addition to you, the PM? List others in the leadership role.
- What is the potential impact on the live system if the change is implemented?
- What is potential impact on the go-live date, if any?

- What would post-live maintenance requirements be?
- What would potential impact on your budget be?
- How will change, if approved, impact the overall scope of project?
- What is the quality of the tasks performed when pushed too quickly against a deadline?

There are many reasons why projects can fail. Table 6.1 summarizes this well and provides some of the more common and frequently seen risks (Carlos, n.d.).

TABLE 6.1
Reasons Why Projects Fail

Problem	Cause	Risk
Poorly managed	Undefined objectives and goals	Lack of management commitment
Lack of a solid project plan	Lack of user input	Lack of organizational support
Centralized proactive management initiatives to combat project risk	Enterprise management of budget resources	Provides universal templates and documentation
Poorly defined roles and responsibilities	Inadequate or vague requirements	Stakeholder conflict
Team weaknesses	Unrealistic timeframes and tasks	Competing priorities
Poor communication	Insufficient resources (funding and personnel)	Business politics
Poorly defined roles and responsibilities	Inadequate or vague requirements	Stakeholder conflict
Team weaknesses	Unrealistic timeframes and tasks	Competing priorities
Poor communication	Insufficient resources (funding and personnel)	Business politics
Overruns of schedule and cost	Estimates for cost and schedule are erroneous	Lack of prioritization and project management
Scope creep	No change control process	Meeting end user expectations
Ignoring project warning signs	Inadequate testing processes	Bad decisions

Adapted from Carlos (n.d.).

The Pareto Principle

As noted in Table 6.1, there are many reasons why projects (both simple and complex) fail; the list is only a partial list. One way to look at this is to focus on most common reasons a project might fail using the Pareto principle. This principle is called the 80/20 rule, meaning that the most common reasons a project might fail can be that 20% of the defects cause 80% of the problems; therefore, a good rule is to focus 80% of your time on the 20% of the work that is really important (Reh, n.d.). If the items and tasks listed in Table 6.1 are closely monitored, there is a good chance there will be few issues—this process of monitoring but not understanding lessons learned from previous projects is a much needed and a huge benefit of the monitor and control process.

Summary of Tools to Monitor and Control

Table 6.2 summarizes the tools and the chapters where found, which correlate with the phases of the project life cycle where the documents would be developed. By way of review, each chapter also includes a discussion of the application processes.

   As previously discussed, the documents needed to monitor and control the project were designed and planned in previous phases, then applied during the implementation phase as the process of monitor and control is also initiated. It is very important that all tasks are monitored; if not using the documents provided, it will be important to at least develop some way to track and monitor all items during the implementation phases.

BENEFITS AND PROCESS
OF CHANGE CONTROL

No one likes change. As discussed in Chapter 4, many resist change at all costs, especially if it is a big change such as the implementation of the electronic health record (EHR). With the implementation of a large project such as an EHR, it will change many things including

TABLE 6.2
Summary of Tools Needed to Monitor and Control With Location

Process	Tool	Chapter Where Found
Scope	Scope tool	3
Charter	Charter tool	3
Project timeline	Example	3
Gap analysis	Example	3
Stakeholder analysis	Stakeholder analysis tool	3
SMART objectives	SMART objective tool	3
WBS	WBS tool	4
SOW	No tool	4
CPM	CPM tool	4
Tracking—Network diagram	Network diagram tool	4
Budget	Budget tool	4
Risk	Risk tool	4
Change management	Change tracking log	4
Weekly status meetings	Meeting tool	4
Project deliverables	Deliverables tool	4
Kick-off meeting	PowerPoint presentation	4
RACI	RACI tool	4
Implementation checklist	Checklist tool	5
Status report	Report tool	5
Change request	Change request tool	5
Communication plan	Communication plan tool	5

CPM, critical path method; RACI, responsible, accountable consulted, informed;
SOW, statement of work; WBS, work breakdown structure.
From Sipes (2014).

workflows, where to find things and how to complete a task. Smaller changes such as evaluation of an improvement process from a single project a DNP completed may not see as much resistance to the new ideas and change. Depending on the change, there typically is resistance, and the larger the change, the more the resistance. During large EHR implementations, there may even be resignations as people do not want to learn new processes or tasks or even feel threatened that their lower level skills will be exposed. An example of the change tracking log can be found in Chapter 4; the change request form can be found in Chapter 5.

QUALITY CONTROL—ROOT CAUSE ANALYSIS

The process of plan, do, check act (PDCA) is a familiar process used when assessing and tracking project tasks and deliverables. Historically, Deming in the 1950s proposed that "... industrial processes should be analyzed and measured to identify sources of variations that cause products to deviate from customer requirements" (Aversion, 1998, p.1). He recommended that business processes be placed in a continuous feedback loop so that managers can identify and change the parts of the process that need improvements.

Although the quality control process of analyzing the root causes was developed for businesses and industry including engineering, the process is viewed as providing a standardized means of monitoring projects of any size. PDCA is defined here; organizations may vary the process to only three tasks—PDA—plan, do, act. The PDCA acronym is:

- **PLAN**: Design or revise business process components to improve results
- **DO**: Implement the plan and measure its performance
- **CHECK**: Assess the measurements and report the results to decision makers
- **ACT**: Decide on changes needed to improve the process

Deming's PDCA cycle (Figure 6.1) reflects a continuous, ongoing cycle. Monitoring the implementation of any project will benefit from

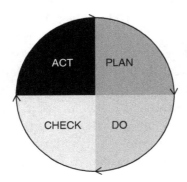

FIGURE 6.1 Deming's PDCA Cycle—Continuous, Ongoing Cycle From Aversion (1998).

TABLE 6.3
PDCA Tool

Plan	Identify the problem; conduct a gap analysis
Do	Analyze the problem; use root cause analysis; implement solutions
Check	Evaluate solutions
Act	If solutions worked, standardize and implement

Adapted from Sipes (2014).

an ongoing and continuous evaluation of how the different aspects are being implemented, where there may be gaps in the process, implementing corrections, and then rechecking the process again (Table 6.3).

Quality management or control requires that tasks be continually monitored and all project documents updated with information sent to all team members and stakeholders—everyone who has a part in the project. It includes such components as budgets, costs, project plan, scope document, testing, metrics, changes and change control, and risks to name a few. A more comprehensive list is included in Table 6.1. It is important to remember that project documents are "living documents," which means they need to be monitored closely and updated as needed, with review and approval from the change control board (CCB) as indicated.

Another component of quality or project control assessment is to conduct a review of overall project performance, which means conducting an evaluation of where the project is in terms of on how well the project, project team, PM, and all others, including stakeholders, are meeting the project's goals and objectives in a timely, on-budget manner.

In summary, quality control is "the process of inspecting products to ensure that they meet the required quality standards" (Riley, 2012, para. 2). The main objective of quality control is to ensure that the business is achieving the standards it sets for itself. The method of quality control or management is the process where the quality of completed products are checked for faults. This usually entails the testing of every product or random samples from each batch if it is not feasible to check every item.

Risk Management

As with all monitoring and control processes, all risks must be evaluated for potential negative impact on the overall project. After all tasks have been monitored, assessed, revised, and updated a report needs to be communicated to all participants in the project including stakeholders and sponsors in a timely manner. A partial list of these tasks is listed here:

- Plan revision—change and update all "living" documents and other project tools. The term "living" document refers to a document that is or may be frequently changed.
- Performance assessment—requires ongoing review of performance from team against the timeline meeting deadlines, against meeting budgets, quality performance with defined metrics in order to track. Question to ask, "Is team sacrificing quality to meet deadlines?"
- Define and create reports that include status reports previously discussed as well as summary and dashboard reports that provide a quick overview of a topic.
- Utilization of the risk management tool previously defined.
- Monitor scope and change control to provide updated documents and prevent scope creep.
- Control of human resources can be monitored using a tool or tracking document that clearly defines job roles and responsibilities that were identified during the project planning phase. They need to be reviewed, monitored and controlled during implementations.
- It is important to understand that not all stakeholders should be treated the same—those who have a high impact should be communicated with more frequently; those with low impact can be kept informed.

Another process frequently used when monitoring progress is called "cause mapping" or gap analysis (see Figure 6.2). This can be done using an Excel spreadsheet, which is an excellent tool for capturing the elements of a complete root cause analysis. By changing the way details are documented, a facilitator can improve the entire investigation process. First the problem or gap is identified, a potential cause and

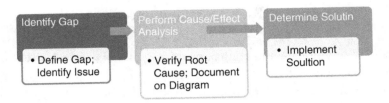

FIGURE 6.2 Cause Mapping
From Sipes (2014).

effect outlined and, finally, a solution is explored. There is an excellent health care map available free if you currently are using or have Excel on your computers. An example can be found in Figure 6.2.

A third process used to break down and analyze an issue is called the fishbone diagram process. "A cause and effect diagram, often called a 'fishbone' diagram, can help in brainstorming to identify possible causes of a problem and in sorting ideas into useful categories. A fishbone diagram is a visual way to look at cause and effect "… and is more structured" … than some other tools that help to identify causes of a problem" (Medicare, 2014, para. 2).

The problem or effect is displayed at the head or mouth of the fish. Possible contributing causes are listed on the smaller "bones" under various cause categories. A fishbone diagram can be helpful in identifying possible causes for a problem that might not otherwise be considered

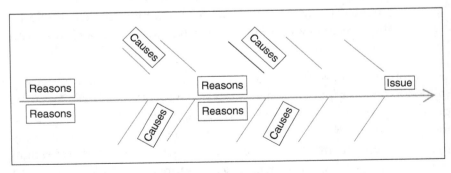

FIGURE 6.3 Root Cause Analysis: Fishbone Example
From Sipes (2014).

TABLE 6.4
Root Cause Analysis Tracking Tool Using Data From Fishbone

Issues and Source (s)	Projected Cause of Issue	Solutions	Risk if Not Mitigated	Assign Owner and Due data
Define the issue and source of cause	What does the group think was the cause based on the investigation?	Recommendations for resolving the problem	High, medium, or low	Who will be responsible for seeing that the issue is resolved?

by directing the team to look at the categories and think of alternative causes. Next, define the real reasons the problem is occurring—what is a symptom of the problem? Include team members who have personal knowledge of the processes and systems involved in the problem or event to be investigated.

After the reasons that may have caused the issues have been determined by the project team, the analysis will need to be documented and tracked. Solutions will be recommended, risks assessed if solutions are not implemented and, finally, critical to the whole process is to assign an owner with due dates. This can be done by developing a tracking tool in Excel such as the example in Table 6.4.

TESTING

Why Do We Need to Conduct Testing?

Testing is required to make sure everything that has been built works the way it was designed. There are many, many different types of testing; they cannot all be completed before a full system "goes live." In the case of a very large EHR implementation, random or selected testing is completed. With smaller applications the entire application can be tested.

Some of the more common terms associated with testing that you may be familiar with include:

- Unit testing—where the "unit" being developed is tested during the building process
- Integration testing—these are tests completed to make sure the "unit" or application works with other units or applications; that is, that it integrates well and does not cause problems

- System testing—a larger testing process to make sure it not only works with some of the applications but works across the system. For example, do medication orders not only work well within the order placement functionality but do the orders flow to all of the areas where an order is needed?
- Acceptance testing—this type of testing is done by the end users; those who will actually be using the application or system to make sure it meets all expectations

Again there are many types of testing such as load testing where many users are asked to complete a function such as entering orders at the same time to see if the system slows down or even fails during a peak use time. Another type of testing is usability testing where an end users works with the new system to determine how easy it is to use. There are many resources on the web that can provide additional information.

SUMMARY

This chapter on monitoring and controlling the project explains the process and the primary objectives of the process, and provides a list of some of the activities that need to be accomplished congruously and ongoing. There is discussion of how to manage new work that might be discovered as well as a discussion of benefits to monitoring. Most importantly, there is a discussion of why projects fail. By understanding what lessons and reasons for failure have been found in other projects, it should help to manage expectations with the current project. Quality control methods are discussed with examples of tools that can be used to monitor quality or suggestions for creating your own tools, listing the key elements that need to controlled. Finally, a summary of why testing is critically needed is provided, including a discussion of some of the most common terms.

REFERENCES

Arveson, P. (1998). The Deming cycle. Retrieved from Balanced Scorecard Institute website: https://balancedscorecard.org/Resources/Articles-White-Papers/The-Deming-Cycle

Carlos, T. (n.d.). *Reasons why projects fail*. Retrieved from www.projectsmart.co.uk

Medicare. (2104). *How to use the fishbone tool for root cause analysis.* Retrieved from www.cms.gov/Medicare/Provider-Enrollment-and Certification/QAPI/ downloads/ FishboneRevised.pdf

Reh, J. (n.d.). *Pareto's principle—The 80/20 rule; how the 80/20 rule can help you be more effective.* Retrieved from http://management.about.com

Riley, J. (2012). *Q&A—Explain what is involved in quality control.* Retrieved from http://www.tutor2u.net

Root Cause Analysis Software: Excel tools. Retrieved fromwww.thinkreliability .com/excel-tools.aspx

Sipes, C. (2014). PDCA Table and tool. Adapted from root cause analysis software: excel tools. Retrieved from www. thinkreliability.com/excel-tools. aspx

CHAPTER 7

Closing the Project—Phase 5

LEARNING OBJECTIVES

Upon completion of this chapter, the reader will be able to:

1. Define three processes of the closing phase
2. Discuss three tasks to be accomplished during the closing phase
3. Discuss the value of analyzing lessons learned at the close of the project
4. Discuss when the closing functions should be implemented

OUTLINE

- Key Terms
- Verification Audit
- Review of Final Deliverables
- Lessons Learned
- Final Report
- Transition of Project Documents and Plans
- Final Analysis and Debriefing
- Formal Acceptance

KEY TERMS

Closing	Review of deliverables
Debrief	Transition
Lessons learned	Verification audit

Closing can be a conflict between the very busy times on the project and moving on to something different, even another project. Whether it is an internal or external project, you must have met the constraints discussed in earlier chapters that were defined for the project. If it is an internal project closing, you must seamlessly transition the project into the company's normal operations. For external projects such as a small project (wedding) or larger project (work related), check formal documents to make sure all deadlines and budgets have been met. Final delivery of the product should be reviewed to make sure it meets the needs and expectations of the organization (Definition of the Closing Process Group in Project, p. 1).

During the closing phase, the tasks that need to be completed include debriefing the team, transitioning all of the appropriate documentation and project history, as well as transitioning all activities back to those who will own, support, and maintain the activity. The primary objective of the closing and transition processes is to obtain formal acceptance of the completed project by the project champion and key stakeholders if indicated. The transition and closing documents are discussed more in detail with examples later in this chapter (Closing Process Group, p.1).

VERIFICATION AUDIT

This audit is a report that summarizes that the products purchased at the beginning of the project were received and working correctly. In addition, these audits should have been conducted throughout the controlling phase of the project. Anything unexpected or out of scope will need to be discussed with leadership and approved with sign-off during this audit.

Sign-Off With Leadership

The final sign-off with leadership validates that there is agreement with the products purchased, the functionality and user acceptance testing (UAT), change requests approved, and all other items listed in the

TABLE 7.1
Verification Audit Document

Verification Audit Task/Product	Owner	Signature/Sponsor/Date
Products (purchased list)		
Functionality/User acceptance testing – Can product be used/function as designed? – Does it meet business needs?		
Change requests approved		
Other tasks from scope document		
Does final project meet success measures outlined in scope document?		
Were all requirements outlined in project plan met?		

From Sipes (2014).

scope document. The report is also shared with all leadership and sponsors and any other businesses involved in the project to provide input and verify that all tasks and outcomes of the project were met (Table 7.1).

REVIEW OF FINAL DELIVERABLES

The project manager (PM) must review responses and determine if final sign-off is acceptable. If not, then a meeting needs to be scheduled with all involved—leadership, sponsors, end users—to determine how best to resolve all and any issues to make it acceptable. It should include review of documents, including risk, change, budget, constraints, and assumptions documents. Specifically, the budget needs to be checked with the key person responsible for the overall budget, including each line item reviewed against original estimates; after this has been completed satisfactorily the budget must be signed off.

All documents listed in the scope and charter documents must be reviewed and discussed with key stakeholders and sponsors to make sure all tasks and processes have been reviewed and completed.

Other key documents that need to be reviewed and signed off during this meeting include the work breakdown structure (WBS) and Gantt chart.

LESSONS LEARNED

What Are Lessons Learned?

Lessons learned is a term frequently used by anyone completing a project—it is time to review, collect, and document information regarding how things went and what can be improved for the next project as well as getting feedback from everyone involved in the project. This is set up as a meeting where it is expected that everyone will be in attendance and contribute to the final assessment. Things that need to be improved upon will be documented and assigned an owner in case there is a need for further resolution.

The outcome of this meeting is to prepare a final report for leadership and stakeholders. The lessons-learned session is usually set up in a meeting or conference room. All who have been involved in the project will be invited to provide comment. One way to do this is to go around the table and have everyone share his or her insights while minutes are being recorded.

Another more confidential and productive way to collect this information is to send out meeting invitations to those who wish to be included in the evaluation process and have them come to an open room where large sheets of paper are put up around the room. The large Post-its will have various topics listed at the top. Then attendees write comments on sticky notes and place them under the topic of choice (see Table 7.2).

After everyone has had a chance to provide input, collect and tabulate the data and prepare the report. Other objectives of the lessons-learned function are to:

- Define additional work that needs to be done
- Determine if there are other changes that need to be made to the project, its processes, or methodology
- Define customer satisfaction with the deliverable and value and benefits of the project
- Review the quality and performance of the project and teams

TABLE 7.2
Lessons Learned Process Example

- **Topic:** Functionality of clinical documentation
  - It was great!
  - It did not function as advertised—it did not do XXXXX
  - It would be better if.....
  - XXX is missing
- **Topic:** Med order process
  - Med ordering did not show correct times
  - Too many clicks to get to the area to enter orders
  - Sign-off function did not work well

From Sipes (2014).

It will be interesting to review the information collected as the report is prepared. An important process during lessons learned is to have all project team members involved in preparing the final report so they can review the comments.

When all documentation is completed a final report will be prepared for leadership and stakeholders. A summary of tasks completed and outcomes of the project includes preparation of the documents including the final report, delivery of all working documents, preparation of the final presentation, and a documented transition plan with formal hand-off and knowledge transfer with owners identified. A review of the critical success factors for the project and outcome of the meeting will need to be documented as well (Project Management Closing—Best Practices, pp. 1–5).

FINAL REPORT

The final report should provide detail about the project and members of the organization who were involved in the project, if applicable. The report should be prepared as a document with consideration that the person reading it may not be familiar with the project. They should be able to read the report and know the "who" involved and at what level, what was done, how it was done, and why the project was needed.

The content will need to be clear, concise, and consistent and contain meaningful information that aligns with the scope documents. If the organization has a standard format for documentation, that must be used. One goal for the report is to include notation that there were tangible deliverables that were clear, insightful, on time, and within budget that were outlined in the project charter.

The basic outline for the document should follow the project life cycle in terms of what happened in each phase of the project and focus on:

- Background of needs
- Project expectations that were consistent with scope
- List of deliverables defined in the project charter
- Preparation of the final report that includes past reports
- Review of potential content of the final report with a project steering team, or other key stakeholder who has been supportive of the project, if there is one.

An example of the final report document is provided in Table 7.3.

The final report will be presented as one formal, professional document with all additional documents added as appendices and noted in the table of contents. It will be important to include all documents bound

TABLE 7.3
Final Report Document

Final Report—Date of Report	Project Manager (Include Who Prepared the Report if Designated)
Title Page: (Client name, location, project title)	
Table of Contents	
Executive Summary: (Organization, purpose, project objective, main outcomes, key recommendations)	
Background and Objectives: (Organization, project objectives, reason for project, issues and documented need, expected results)	
Approach: (Detail scope of project, implementation process with tasks—can include WBS as appendix and refer to it)	
Findings: (Summary of findings—refer to WBS—add other appendices with references to them)	
Recommendations: (Based on key findings and issues)	
Conclusion: (Summarize/ discuss approach and processes used, project objectives, issues with resolutions)	
Appendices	

From Sipes (2014).

together as one or in a notebook. It is difficult, appears disorganized, and is more time consuming if there are many separate documents to review.

TRANSITION OF PROJECT DOCUMENTS AND PLANS

Transition Plans

Why do you need a transition plan or hand-off? Project transition is also referred to a knowledge transfer because it involves educating the new owners of the project tasks on the key elements of the project, what went well, and what might need further work or revisions. Closing a project includes a number of activities and tasks that need to be completed by the PM as well as the project team. A number of the project closing documents will have been completed as discussed earlier; now it is time to review to make sure everything has been completed and a plan is in place for archiving the documents and as well as the formal handoff to the new owners of tasks that might need to be competed yet or maintained. In addition to developing the project closing documents, which will include the milestones and verification audit, you will also need to develop a transition and hand-off plan.

The transition plan is important in that it will provide the stakeholders, leadership, and team members with information on the project completion and transition back to anyone who might continue with other phases or optimization of the same project. The final documents should be kept in a file where all management documents are kept. Information and documents included in the transition plan will be the transfer of any outstanding work that remains that will be completed in the next phase or go to information technology support or a designee to oversee any maintenance that might be needed.

The final meeting should be set up and include the project sponsor and stakeholders if appropriate, and others from the project team. Tasks include preparing an agenda including the intent of a meeting to review the lists of all documents that will be turned over to the new owners, and key highlights of what transpired during the four or five different phases of the project. It is also important to emphasize the turnover and handoff to the new owners who will formally sign-off at the conclusion of the meeting, which indicates they understand the project has ended from your perspective.

The transition documents should include:

- Final report
- A list of all presentations related to the project
- A list of files, documents, reports
- A list of all deliverables including documentation of processes and change reports
- Maintenance and system requirements going forward
- Identification of any additional work that needs to be completed as well as all documents that have been completed, including status reports, risk management plans, and other documented tasks; create an "open issues and incomplete tasks" report

These documents should be prepared in both paper and electronic formats. The project sponsors will indicate where they want the documents archived (Project Closure, pp. 1–3).

FINAL ANALYSIS AND DEBRIEFING

The final analysis and debriefing is an important step—overlooked by many as too time consuming. But this process provides an opportunity to review the project's successes and failures. It also provides opportunities to add success measures that are not already defined. During this meeting it will be important to review the outcome and value of the project, review additional work if needed, review deficiencies, recommend changes for processes that did not work, and review the quality of the project and overall satisfaction of the project.

FORMAL ACCEPTANCE

What is formal acceptance? Not only is preparing all final documents during the closing phase an important task, but also getting formal and final sign-off from the project sponsors is a must. When this process is complete it indicates the sponsors have reviewed all of the documentation provided, have discussed and understand the issues and recommendations presented, and now accept the final report with a signature.

TABLE 7.4
Project Modifications During Project

Original Milestones From Scope	Modification Status	Final Milestones
		Agreement:
		Sign-off date:

From Sipes (2014).

The report should include a review of the key milestones from the original scope and charter documents, the due dates for those and whether they were adjusted and how they were met. If there were revisions of the milestones, those will need to be included in the report (see Table 7.4). It will be critical to obtain a signature to verify the review of the documents and activities, and formally conclude the meeting.

SUMMARY

The closing phase of the project indicates the project has been completed and now is ready for hand off and transition to the original organization or party, whoever originally requested the project. This chapter introduces the final processes necessary to formally and legally close out a project and includes the description of the verification audit with an example of a verification audit tool. It also provides discussion of project deliverables, lessons-learned processes and a lessons-learned tool to use during the final meeting.

A description of elements needed in the final report as well as the final report tool are provided, along with the discussion of what should be included in the transition plan and transition documents. The final three topics include the final analysis and debriefing, formal acceptance, and a project modification during the project. A PM will use any or all of these tools. Many of the tools were developed, altered, and revised for use on many different and varied projects, both large and small, from very large to much smaller organizations and health systems.

REFERENCES

Closing Process Group—Project Management Resources; http://www.villanovau.com/resources/project-management/pmbok-closing-process-group/#.VdYeOLJViko; p 1.

The Closing Process Group—Bright Hub Project Management www.brighthubpm.com

Project Management: Closing—the Best Practices (2010). http://www.virtualprojectconsulting.com/project-management-closure-best-practice/. p 1.

Project Closure—Mastering Project Management www.mastering-project-management.com/project-closure.html. p 1.

Application of Project Management Concepts and Tools

CHAPTER 8

Case Studies: Applying Project Management Concepts and Tools

LEARNING OBJECTIVES

Upon completion of this chapter, the reader will be able to:

1. Discuss two project management tasks a nurse practitioner (NP) would need in practice
2. List three project management skills a chief nursing informatics officer (CNIO) would use
3. Discuss three project management skills a nurse executive would need vs. those a nurse manager would need
4. Discuss the project management tools and processes a clinical nurse specialist (CNS) might use to start up a new clinic
5. Describe three of the nine steps a doctor of nursing practice (DNP) will take to develop a project in the doctorate program that is required for graduation

OUTLINE

- Key Terms
- How the APN and DNP Roles Would Use Project Management Concepts
- APN and DNP Roles—Where Concepts Apply

KEY TERMS

Advanced practice nurse (APN)
Chief nursing informatics officer
  (CNIO)
Chief nursing officer (CNO)
Clinical nursing specialist (CNS)

Doctor of nursing practice (DNP)
Informatics nurse specialist (INS)
Nurse executive (NE)
Nurse practitioner (NP)

A number of students have said that, "one thing you don't learn in nursing school is project management" (personal communication, November 11, 2014). Or do you? While nurses may not receive formal training on business topics, there are many skills they do learn that can help them conceive and manage projects in the workplace. For example, the nursing process provides an ideal background for using project management techniques. The nursing process incorporates a systematic method of assessment, diagnosis, planning, implementation, and evaluation. Project management is very similar and encompasses comparable procedures and processes.

There are many roles the advanced practice nurse (APN) can assume given the opportunity to develop knowledge and skills needed for a particular role or job. The intent of this chapter is to suggest and demonstrate by example how different tasks associated with the different roles the APN will assume can be applied in practice. There is the belief that nurses do not or will not use project management concepts in practice; however, there are many terms that are consistent in both project management and nursing practice, such as the nursing process. The different case studies presented here will add clarity to project management terms when the overlap in semantics is noted.

Literature suggests that APNs today are not adequately prepared for advanced leadership roles, which adds to higher levels of turnover in these positions (Staggers et al., 2002). One of the skills identified in the literature is referred to as informatics competencies, of which project management is a foundational concept, although the skills that come under this umbrella today have been used by nurses in a variety of ways for a number of years (www.ala.org/ala, 2015). For example, having the ability to log on and document in a computer where the computer is the primary mode of entering patient data has been a function nurses have assumed for a number of years. Historically, nursing education did not include informatics competencies; thus, current managers, administrators, or nurse executives (NEs) may not be adequately prepared to use or lead change in the use of health information technology (HIT) (Westra & Delaney, 2008).

HOW THE APN AND DNP ROLES WOULD USE PROJECT MANAGEMENT CONCEPTS

National nursing organizations' leadership is beginning to define skills needed in many nursing roles; some examples of APN roles and application of skills that will be needed can be found here. One such example is from the American Organization of Nurse Executives (AONE). The organization's last review of NE competencies occurred in 2005; AONE supports that "management's role is pivotal in organizational transformation using EHRs and other HITs" (AONE, 2008, p. 804). The AONE's Nursing Executive Competencies lists skills in communication and business skills, all of which overlap with leadership competencies. Another national organization, Healthcare Information and Management Systems Society (HIMSS, 2013), states that "Nursing leaders must have computer and informatics knowledge and skills to work with other disciplines."

APN AND DNP ROLES—WHERE CONCEPTS APPLY

There are eight examples and case studies of different roles an APN will need to utilize project management concepts and tools in his or her practice. The roles include the nurse administrator as an NE or nurse manager, a nurse practitioner (NP), a clinical nursing specialist (CNS), an informatics nurse specialist (INS), a chief nursing informatics officer (CNIO), a chief nursing officer (CNO), and a doctor of nursing practice (DNP) student in the final practicum before graduation.

Case Study—Nurse Administrator

Nurse Executive

Becky R. has a master's of science in nursing (MSN) and is the new NE for ABC Medical Center, a 35-bed, medical–surgical department. She is in charge of 55 RNs and patient care technicians (PCTs). Becky was just recently promoted from the nurse manager position to the NE position. In this position she brings a number of skills she acquired as the nurse manager but also is expected to have additional leadership skills including:

- Ability to manage finances—cost containment
- Provide oversight for operational and capital budgets
- Determine cost–benefit analysis, unit budget control measures,
- Understand financial resource procurement and develop monitoring plans
- Develop and set measureable objectives
- Identify key stakeholders for projects
- Prepare reports, metrics, tables, graphs charts, and dashboard reports
- Propose actions, build on past lessons learned
- Monitor outcomes
- Develop and understand workflow processes
- Manage time
- Be consistent; have consistent processes
- Provide and understand organizational governance
- Monitor quality improvement

In Becky's previous job as the nurse manager, she had the opportunity to take two project manager (PM) courses at the university where she became more proficient in such skills as developing communication plans, communicating with organizational leadership through report writing, and attending meetings where she also learned to work well with group process. She learned to develop change management plans and by doing so utilized the change process to become more knowledgeable in team building and managing conflict, while providing resolutions and managing resources; she became more computer literate as well. All of the skills she developed aided in her promotion to NE (Chapters 3 and 4).

One of the conditions of her promotion was that she would need to take further courses to learn how to manage finances—cost containment, provide oversight for operational and capital budgets, determine cost–benefit analysis, unit budget control measures, understand financial resource procurement, and develop monitoring plans that also includes monitoring quality improvement (Chapters 4 to 6).

The CNO at this organization has the skills and expertise that she has developed over the years in order to get promoted, so she will initially take on a partial role for managing the finances and all other budgets while Becky learns how to do this. Becky has some knowledge that she had to develop as a nurse manager but not at the level now required in the NE position. The CNO recommends that since Becky already has her MSN that she complete the Nursing Informatics Certificate courses at the online university where she will have the opportunity to gain further project management skills in managing finances and budgets (Chapter 4). The CNO also noted that Becky will need to understand and develop workflows, develop box diagrams, and monitor and control for quality improvement (Chapters 4 to 6). Becky agrees and arranges to take the courses as they work to establish a timeline for her to complete these goals.

Nurse Manager

Ruth S., a newly graduated MSN, is the nurse manager who reports to Becky and as a new nurse manager is required to learn how to plan and schedule staff to adequately cover a dynamic and frequently changing work environment. She has also been asked to manage the budget for the unit, something she will need to learn as she has not done this before. Ruth has had an introduction to the basic skills in her master's program but not to the extent she will need to perform her role functions well.

There are other competencies she will need to learn as a manager and, just as her predecessor, will take the same two PM courses at the university where she will develop skills such as developing communication plans, learn how to communicate with organizational leadership through report writing, and attendance at meetings where she will learn more about the group process (Chapter 4). She will learn to develop change management plans and by doing so will learn how to utilize the change process to become more knowledgeable in team building and managing conflict, as well as provide resolutions and manage resources; she became more computer literate as well (Chapters 3 and 4).

Ruth is not well versed in finance so Becky, who promoted her, initially will take on this task until Ruth becomes more conformable with the process (Chapter 4). With oversight from Becky, Ruth will need to review and validate how to assign tasks, as well as delegate, deal with conflict, and assess and prioritize timelines (Chapter 4). Becky also suggested that Ruth work with other peers who have expertise in data collection and analysis, understand how to collect data, analyze and prepare reports for the CNO and NE, define the metrics leadership will require, and review outcomes (Chapters 3 and 4). Ruth will learn how to do other tasks as she takes the courses in project management. Other tasks include the ability to:

- Develop objectives for both short-term and long-term goals (Chapter 4)
- Develop and plan a and b options (Chapter 4)
- Take action and know when to delegate (Chapter 5)
- Define what processes need to be in place (Chapters 3 and 4)
- Determine how to monitor and control (Chapter 6)

Ruth has also been told that the ABC Medical Center will be implementing a new system to document and track nursing standards. She will need to work with information technology (IT) to implement the system and ensure the system for implementation of standards is in place, including a method for documenting employees exceeding or failing to meet standards, (Chapters 4 and 5).

Ruth realizes that she will be very busy at least for her first 6 months in the new job and works with Becky to establish a timeline for all of the new tasks including her school work (Chapter 4).

Case Study—Nurse Practitioner

Jill O. is a master's level student who has completed her core courses in an NP graduate program and now needs to develop a project for the two practicums she will need to complete before she can graduate. Jill has found a mentor at the St. Louis Medical Center who will help guide her through her first practicum. Her mentor is an MSN with project management experience and has been managing the department that Jill will be working in to complete her practicum. The first week in the department, Jill's mentor asked her to review some data she has regarding patients with higher than average wait times to be seen by medical personnel in a specific department and to look for specific issues such as lack of resources including personnel, computers, or other issues that might be contributing to the wait times. Based on her own practice and the courses she has just completed, Jill knows what needs to be done when completing the history and physical assessments.

Jill and her mentor put together a preliminary project plan for her practice that the two of them will present to her practicum instructor. In the practicum, the course guidelines require that she first develop a scope document and project charter that outline measureable objectives and deliverables for her project (Chapter 3). After the meeting with the instructor and mentor it was determined that she will need to revise her objectives to be more specific and include who will be responsible for each task with due dates and update her work plan (Chapter 4). Jill will oversee the data collection and analysis and determine how the reports should be presented to the key stakeholders (Chapter 6).

In the work plan, Jill will develop the process for who, what, where, and when the status meetings will be held and how action items will be resolved (Chapter 5). Jill will need to develop a risk mitigation plan outlining the risks to specific patient populations that are put on a wait list and to develop a plan for how certain patient groups will be prioritized (Chapter 4). She will also need to develop recommendations to resolve any issues regarding the lack of resources, who would be scheduling patients, and a plan to add more training (Chapter 4). At this point, Jill does not have the authority to control and manage the budget; therefore, her mentor will complete the actual task but teach Jill how she might do this in the future (Chapter 4). Jill will conduct the resource assessment and prepare a report with recommendations for more personnel and computers as well as training (Chapter 5) that she will present to her mentor and key stakeholders.

Case Study—Clinical Nurse Specialist

Cindy J. has just graduated from the master's program with her CNS and is now preparing to set up her diabetes clinic in the Des Moines Medical Center. She will be working with a peer, Kathy, who has

7 years' experience in independent practice in the clinic but now has asked Cindy to join her practice. Cindy is hesitant, telling Kathy she knows nothing about setting up and running a clinic, that she has only managed a group of her own patients.

Kathy tells her not to worry, that she has management experience as a PM, which she gained while in another practice with someone who had a lot of project management experience, and that she will help Cindy using project management tools she also used in the past. Cindy also keeps the course text she used in her practicum that has examples of project management tools to use with examples of how to use each of them.

Kathy tells Cindy that first she will need to put together a plan for how she wants the clinic to run and suggests she use a Gantt chart (Chapter 4) that will define the days, who will be on what days for all of the clinic employees, and all of the different tasks that will be needed in the clinic. Later, after Cindy has completed the chart and assigned different tasks, she will formalize content from the chart into a weekly schedule that will be used permanently after the clinic is set up. Next she will need to develop a scope document (Chapter 3) that will define exactly what they will do and not do in the clinic and a charter (Chapter 3) for the clinic that will define the mission, levels of authority, and other key stakeholders. Cindy will also need to develop a risk management plan (Chapter 4) that will outline how risks will be managed, strategies for mitigating risks, and a responsibility matrix (Chapter 4) that will outline owners of the different responsibilities in the clinic. Kathy tells Cindy that she will manage the budget for now until Cindy gets up to speed, then show her how to set up and manage the budget (Chapter 4). Kathy has already set up a communication plan but asks that Cindy review and revise it now that the clinic is growing (Chapter 5). Cindy will need to set up status meetings after first determining how often they will be needed and the format that should be used (Chapter 5), also to determine how they will monitor and control all that is happening in the new clinic (Chapter 6).

Case Study—Informatics Nurse Specialist

June S. has just assumed the INS role. She recently moved into the role from that of an RN where she worked in the emergency department and completed her MSN with a specialty in nursing informatics. Her role is to help nurses and other health care providers by facilitating the entry of patient data into the new electronic medical record (EMR) once it is implemented. June's training to support the EMR implementation will start with a review and analysis of the workflow process for clinical documentation the nurses will be using on the medical–surgery floors of the MC Medical Center. She understands that she will need to interview the nurses to conduct a needs assessment of the current state—"what is" workflows—then help them to understand the future state or "what will be" workflows, just as she did for her graduate practicum (Chapters 3 and 4).

After she has completed the needs assessment, June will develop goals and objectives for the clinical documentation application implementation of the EMR. She will work with Susan, the CNIO, to provide the information Susan will need as she develops the scope and charter documents necessary for final approval of the EMR implementation (Chapter 3). June will also be responsible for developing the work breakdown structure (WBS) for the different tasks and team members after the team has been interviewed and hired for this project (Chapter 3). Once the WBS has been developed and approved, June will need to develop a responsibility matrix (RACI [responsible, accountable, consulted, informed]) tracking document, and establish the team meeting structure (Chapter 3).

June understands she will have to pick a number of INS roles as the medical center starts to design, plan, and implement the new EHR that everyone is talking about. Susan, the CNIO, has suggested several roles and responsibilities that she would like June to assume as soon as the final project charter and scope are agreed on by leadership.

Case Study—Chief Nurse Informatics Officer

Susan P. is the CNIO for MC Medical Center, which is in the process of designing and implementing the new EMR system they will be implementing institution-wide and at some of the outlying clinics within the next year. She has experience developing financial plans and the budget to support the EMR but is also working with the CFO to make sure that she has developed a budget to cover all beyond the clinical application implementations (Chapter 4).

Her role as the leader requires that she provide support for the PM who has been selected and provide oversight for the project scope, objectives, and identify resources for each proposed application, system, or enhancement (Chapter 4). Susan will ensure that the principles and concepts of project management are used for the implementation of information systems (Chapter 5), which will provide a framework that demonstrates a step-wise process and collaborates on oversight with other leaders to ensure that testing plans are developed, implemented, and evaluated at every phase of system implementations (HIMSS, 2013, p. 2; see Chapters 4 to 6). Many of the processes and roles will be delegated to others such as the nursing mangers, INS, and those who have the required skill sets for a specific job function.

Susan will work collaboratively with the interdisciplinary leaders to establish short- and long-term goals and the specific implementation plans for clinical information systems that have been purchased for MC Medical Center. She will work to incorporate her goals into the organizations goals that include the following:

- Improve the clinical quality, safety, and operational integrity of clinical information systems (CIS)
- Integrate quality improvement and regulatory standards into the CIS to maximize the capability of the clinical data warehouse for quality, research, and evidence-based practice activities
- Work to develop, implement, and evaluate systems and data, and processes that complement the overall system for performance improvement
- Work to evaluate factors related to safety, outcomes, effectiveness, cost, and social impact when supporting the development and implementation of practice innovations
- Work with the CFO on the budget to develop methods to secure appropriate fiscal and human resources to accomplish the work/goals
- Ensure that effective systems exist and are maintained where data collection and information systems are utilized to improve patient care

Susan has many of the skills and knowledge required of a CNIO listed here but she did not feel comfortable completing a budget by herself that also included the implementation of a major EHR for the organization as well as several outlying clinics. The CFO is working with her to finalize the needed budgets and will continue to provide oversight for all of the budgets.

Case Study—Chief Nursing Officer

Camille R. has just been appointed as the new CNO with the Medical Center expansion and reorganization. The Medical Center is expanding nursing roles and encouraging more nurses to become involved in administration and leadership where the roles and responsibilities of nurses are expanding and taking on executive positions, which are a crucial part of reorganization. With this expansion and promotion, Camille has been asked to attend an executive development program that will provide her with the knowledge and competencies that these executive positions require to become a successful NE. As the CNO, she realizes she will play a critical role in hospital reorganization that requires a diverse set of executive leadership and professional competencies (Batcheller, 2011).

In her new role, she reviews her job description and in a meeting with the Medical Center chief executive officer (CEO) goes over each of the functions she is expected to assume as the CNO. She discusses how her role is to develop, maintain, and evaluate an environment of excellence that supports the professional nurse and other nursing care providers. She further discusses how she will be responsible and accountable for the overall management of nursing practice, nursing education and professional development, nursing research, especially the implementation of evidence-based practice, and nursing administration of nursing services.

The CEO asks her to be more specific and list how she will accomplish the high-level responsibilities. Camille discusses how her role in organizational leadership requires that she continue to maintain current knowledge in administrative practice and acquire ongoing leadership development throughout the organization in areas where she has had little experience. She asks the CEO to make specific suggestions on how she might accomplish this, given the Medical Center's reorganization. The CEO also emphasizes that she provide critically important leadership by creating, coordinating, and reinforcing mission, vision, values and expectations that will set new directions in health care, especially since the Medical Center is reorganizing.

The CEO further suggests that she will need more education regarding the budget and will need to take some courses since she will have to:

- Participate in planning and monitoring the budget for specific areas (Chapter 4)

- Participate in the annual resource allocations and other project management and leadership functions (Chapters 3 to 5)
- Collaborate with nursing councils, nursing leaders, interdisciplinary teams, executive officers, and other stakeholders including the nurse directors (Chapters 3 and 5)
- Be responsible for teaching, coaching, mentoring, and challenging all staff to use quality improvement and project management principles by setting expectations and planning, and reviewing quality and operational performance (Chapters 3 to 7)
- Set performance excellence goals and directions in health care through organization-wide strategy mapping (Chapters 3 to 6)
- Review overall performance including all stakeholders; interests and operational performance (Frederickson & Nickitas, 2011; see Chapters 4 and 5)
- Ensure that the nursing services are in alignment with organizational priorities, goals, and objectives (Carriere, Muise, Cummings, & Newburn-Cook, 2009; see Chapters 4 to 6)
- Foster continuous, positive peer review and ongoing leadership development throughout organization

Six months later, Camille has completed two terms at the university where she took the project management courses she needed to acquire the skills she needs for her new role. In her latest one-on-one meeting with her CEO, she states she is feeling much more conformable in the role of CNO.

Case Study—Doctorate of Nursing Practice

Robin K. has been a practicing nurse with an MSN for over 11 years. She is now in the DNP program, has completed all of her core courses, and is now starting her final practicum. She has completed research on the role of the DNP and found that NEs typically practice in a business environment, which requires a skill set that has traditionally not been included in the advanced nursing curriculum. Robin found that the DNP essentials are designed to address this gap in education while maintaining the focus on advanced nursing practice as well as executive management competencies. In her research she found a study that looked at roles of a CNO and how the service provided is better and more advanced when the CNO pursues the DNP degree. The report further noted that practicing CNOs in multiple care settings "perceive the DNP as an appropriate degree for nurse executive roles" (Swanson & Stanton, 2013).

Today it is expected that APNs have technology knowledge, skills, and ability as well as leadership skills such as financial ability and knowledge. Robin has identified a mentor for her project and will focus the project on the implementation and application of evidence to resolve the problem or gap in the problem she has identified.

In her first meeting with her mentor and DNP faculty, they begin to discuss the design of her project, establish a timeline, costs, and other boundaries including measureable objectives of what she intends to accomplish with the project (Chapter 3). They discuss some of the tools she will use to implement and monitor and control the project (Chapters 4 to 6) with the final closing and evaluation of the project that will be reported back to leadership (Chapter 7). Robin's mentor reviews the nine steps the DNP faculty outlined regarding how she will need to complete the development, implementation, and evaluation of her project.

She will first conduct a problem analysis by critically thinking through the gap analysis of the current state/future state analysis or the "what is/what could be." In the first two steps, a needs assessment is completed in order to determine what needs to be done. She will start by reviewing data, interview stakeholders who may have identified the problem, even conduct a focus group, conduct an organizational assessment, including the mission statement, and review any and all data from relevant websites. Robin will need to assess resources she will need on the project including team members with expertise and skills in the areas in which she has limited knowledge, as well as financial and other costs. Will she need to write a grant to obtain other monies? For steps three through six, she will then compile all of this information into formal documents called the scope and charter (Chapter 3). As the design of her project begins to take shape, she will need to continually revise and update it as she obtains more information. She will need to add measureable, specific objectives to the scope document that will set boundaries and time limits for what will be included and what will be out of scope for this project. Lewis (2007) developed the acronym SMART to be used when writing an objective, which stands for specific, measureable, attainable, realistic, and timely. Objectives are clear, realistic, specific, and measureable actions that move the project toward achieving goals and completion (Lewis, 2007). Specific questions to ask when writing objectives include asking the "five Ws" and "H," who, what, where, when, and why, and how (see Chapter 3).

Once her scope and charter have been approved, she will need to develop other documents and will need to monitor and track her project once it has been implemented. These documents include developing:

- Project plan
- Constraints
- RACI
- Network diagram
- Cost–benefit tracking tools
- Budget
- Risk management plan
- Gantt chart
- Timeline
- Communication plan
- Workflow analysis
- WBS
- Change management plan (Chapter 4)

Once all of the steps in the first two phases of project management, design/initiation and planning, have been completed Robin is ready to implement her project. Since Robin is in the DNP program, she will need to submit all of the work and documents described to her institutional review board (IRB) for approval. Although this process is not part of the project management process it is discussed here as an expectation of the DNP program. Since this process does take time, Robin will need to include this in her timeline. Once approval from the IRB is obtained, Robin will need to set up a project kick-off meeting that formalizes the project start (Chapter 4).

Robin has now implemented her project and is constantly tracking the tasks and resources in the project to monitor every step in the implementation to make sure it is on time, within budget, and meeting the specific objectives and timeline. She will need to monitor the scope very closely to make sure there is no scope creep that can cause a project to fail. At this point in the project, she cannot delegate any of the leadership functions to someone else but must be very clear on the direction of the project (Chapter 5 and 6).

As Robin completes the project tasks listed earlier, she begins to formalize the project closure and evaluation dates to include the key stakeholders in a meeting where she will review and summarize the project success and final results. She will also establish the formal sign-off and completion as well as define the transition processes as she transfers knowledge to institutional leadership. Finally, she will conduct a lessons-learned meeting where things that might have gone better are reviewed, documented, and a final formal report is sent to the CEO (Chapter 7).

SUMMARY

This chapter provides examples of how the different APN roles might be utilized, depending on the various organizations. The roles include how project management concepts and tools might be applied in the nurse administrator—NE and nurse manager roles, as well as an NP who is completing her graduate practicum project and a CNS who is setting up her first diabetes clinic. Finally, it includes examples of how the project management concepts and tools will be utilized in a newly promoted CNO or CNIO and the DNP student who is designing and implementing her final graduate project.

REFERENCES

American Organization for Nurse Executives (AONE). (2005). Nurse executive competencies. *Nurse Leader, 3,* 15–21. Retrieved from www.aone.org/aone/pdf/February%20Nurse%20Leader--final%20draft--for%20web.pdf

Association of College & Research Libraries Information Literacy Competency Standards for Higher Education Association of Colleges & Research Libraries. (2015). Framework for information literacy in higher education of interest. Retrieved from www.ala.org/ala/acrl/acrlstandards/informationliteracy-competency.htm#ildef

Batcheller, J. (2011). On-boarding and enculturation of new chief nursing officers. *Journal of Nursing Administration, 41*(5), 235–239. doi:10.1097/NNA.0b013e3182171c6a

Carriere B., Muise M., Cummings G., Newburn-Cook C. (2009). Healthcare succession planning: An integrative review. *Journal of Nursing Administration, 39*(12), 548–555. doi:10.1097/NNA.0b013e3181c18010

Frederickson, K., & Nickitas, D. (2011). Chief nursing officer executive development: A crisis or a challenge? *Nursing Administration Quarterly, 35*(4), 344–353. doi:10.1097/NAQ.0b013e31822f8e5c

Healthcare Information and Management Systems Society (HIMSS). (2013). www.himss.org/Professional Development, Career Services May 2013/ CNIO

Staggers N., Gassert, C. A., & Curran, C. (2002) A Delphi study to determine informatics competencies for nurses at four levels of practice. Nursing Research, *51*, 383–390.

Swanson, M., & Stanton, M. (2013). Chief nursing officers' perceptions of the Doctorate of Nursing Practice degree. *Nursing Forum, 48*(1), 35–44. doi:10.1111/nuf.12003

Westra, B., & Delaney, C., (2008). Informatics competencies for nursing and health care leaders. National Center for Biotechnology Information. *AMIA Annual Symposium Proceedings*, 804–808. Retrieved October 19, 2014 from www.ncbi.nlm.nih.gov

Index

Note: Page numbers followed by *f* and *t* indicate figures and tables, respectively.

CPSIA information can be obtained
at www.ICGtesting.com
Printed in the USA
BVHW052001150319
542828BV00029B/232/P